T0200180

Manual of
Nerve Conduction Study
and Surface Anatomy
for Needle Electromyography

Manual of Nerve Conduction Study and Surface Anatomy for Needle Electromyography

Fourth Edition

HANG J. LEE, MD

Professor
Department of Rehabilitation Medicine
Korea University College of Medicine
Seoul, Korea

Clinical Professor
Department of Physical Medicine and Rehabilitation
University of Medicine and Dentistry of New Jersey
New Jersey Medical School
Newark, New Jersey

JOEL A. DELISA, MD, MS

Professor and Chair
Department of Physical Medicine and Rehabilitation
University of Medicine and Dentistry of New Jersey
New Jersey Medical School
Newark, New Jersey

President & Chief Executive Officer
Kessler Medical Rehabilitation Research and Education Corporation
West Orange, New Jersey

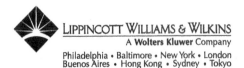

LIPPINCOTT WILLIAMS & WILKINS
A **Wolters Kluwer** Company
Philadelphia • Baltimore • New York • London
Buenos Aires • Hong Kong • Sydney • Tokyo

Acquisitions Editor: Robert Hurley
Developmental Editor: Jenny Kim
Project Manager: Nicole Walz
Senior Production Editor: Michie Shaw, TechBooks
Senior Manufacturing Manager: Ben Rivera
Design coordinator: Holly Reid McLaughlin
Cover and interior design: Mike Pottman
Compositor: TechBooks
Printer: Strategic Content Imaging

© **2005 by LIPPINCOTT WILLIAMS & WILKINS**
530 Walnut Street
Philadelphia, PA 19106 USA
LWW.com

All rights reserved. This book is protected by copyright. No part of this book may be reproduced in any form or by any means, including photocopying, or utilized by any information storage and retrieval system without written permission from the copyright owner, except for brief quotations embodied in critical articles and reviews. Materials appearing in this book prepared by individuals as part of their official duties as U.S. government employees are not covered by the above-mentioned copyright.

Printed in the USA

Library of Congress Cataloging-in-Publication Data

Lee, Hang J.
 Manual of nerve conduction study and surface anatomy for needle electromyography / Hang J. Lee, Joel A. DeLisa.—4th ed.
  p.; cm.
 Rev. ed. of: Manual of nerve conduction velocity and clinical neurophysiology / Joel A. DeLisa ... [et al.]. 3rd ed. c1994 and Surface anatomy for clinical needle electromyography / Hang J. Lee and Joel A. DeLisa. c2000.
 Includes bibliographical references.
 ISBN 0-7817-5821-1 (hardcopy : alk. paper)
 1. Neural conduction—Measurement—Handbooks, manuals, etc.
 2. Somatosensory evoked potentials—Handbooks, manuals, etc.
 3. Electromyography—Handbooks, manuals, etc. I. DeLisa, Joel A.
 II. Lee, Hang J. Surface anatomy for clinical needle electromyography.
 III. Title. IV. Title: Manual of nerve conduction velocity and clinical neurophysiology.
  [DNLM: 1. Muscle, Skeletal—anatomy & histology—Handbooks.
 2. Neural Conduction—Handbooks. 3. Electromyography—methods—Handbooks. 4. Evoked Potentials, Somatosensory—Handbooks.
 WL 39 L478m 2004]
RC349.N48M28 2004
616.8'047547—dc22   2004015993

Care has been taken to confirm the accuracy of the information presented and to describe generally accepted practices. However, the authors, editors, and publisher are not responsible for errors or omissions or for any consequences from application of the information in this book and make no warranty, expressed or implied, with respect to the currency, completeness, or accuracy of the contents of the publication. Application of this information in a particular situation remains the professional responsibility of the practitioner.
The authors, editors, and publisher have exerted every effort to ensure that drug selection and dosage set forth in this text are in accordance with current recommendations and practice at the time of publication. However, in view of ongoing research, changes in government regulations, and the constant flow of information relating to drug therapy and drug reactions, the reader is urged to check the package insert for each drug for any change in indications and dosage and for added warnings and precautions. This is particularly important when the recommended agent is a new or infrequently employed drug.
Some drugs and medical devices presented in this publication have Food and Drug Administration (FDA) clearance for limited use in restricted research settings. It is the responsibility of the health care provider to ascertain the FDA status of each drug or device planned for use in their clinical practice.

21 22 23 24 25

DEDICATION

To my wife, Young, and my children, Edward and Jennifer.
Hang J. Lee

To my trainees, who stimulated me to improve electrodiagnostic teaching.
Joel A. DeLisa

Table of Contents

Part 1

Nerve Conduction Study

CHAPTER 1

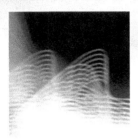

Introduction

Nerve conduction studies are technical procedures used to objectively assess the functional state of the peripheral neuromuscular system. Standardized technical procedures increase the reliability of the studies. The standardized procedures presented in this book represent the consensus of experts who routinely perform nerve conduction studies and whose studies have been published in peer-reviewed journals.

 ## *Basic Nerve Conduction Studies: General Information*

The study of nerve conduction assumes that when a nerve is stimulated electrically a reaction should occur somewhere along the nerve. The reaction of the nerve to stimulation can be monitored with appropriate recording electrodes. Direct recording can be done along sensory or mixed nerves. Indirect recording from a muscle can be used for motor conduction studies. Orthodromic and antidromic conduction can be studied, because stimulus propagation occurs both proximal and distal to the point of stimulation. Orthodromic conduction is the same direction as physiological conduction (e.g., sensory conduction toward the spinal cord and motor conduction away from the spinal cord). Antidromic conduction is propagation in the opposite direction. The time relationship between the stimulus and the response can be displayed, measured, and recorded.

ELECTRODES

Active (recording) and reference electrodes are used. The type of metal surface electrodes used is determined by the type of nerve response being studied.

Motor Response

Peripheral nerves may be stimulated by passing electrical currents through the skin, resulting in a synchronized muscle contraction. When recorded by surface electrodes, this is called the compound muscle action potential (CMAP). Motor responses are recorded over the muscle being studied. The active (recording) electrode (E1) should be placed over the motor point of the muscle so that a clear negative deflection (upward) is recorded when electrostimulation is applied to the nerve supplying that muscle. The reference electrode (E2) should be placed off the muscle on a nearby tendon or bone. Standard recording and reference electrodes are about 1.0 cm in diameter. The surface disc electrodes may be separate discs or fixed 2.0 to 3.0 cm apart in a plastic bar. For standardization or comparisons, E1 and E2 used in CMAP recording should be the same size.

Sensory Response

A compound nerve action potential produced by electrical stimulation of the afferent nerve may be recorded over peripheral sensory nerves in a number of areas. The reference electrode usually is the same type as the recording electrode, and in antidromic studies it is placed distal to the recording electrode. For the orthodromic recording, the reference electrode is placed proximal to the recording

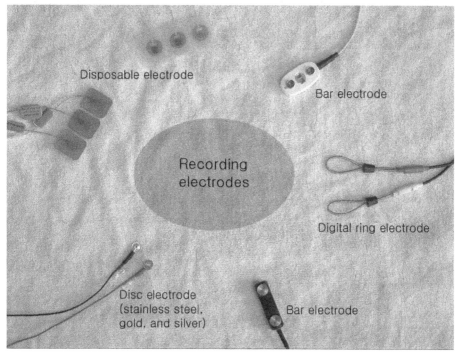

Figure 1-1. *Different types of surface recording electrodes.*

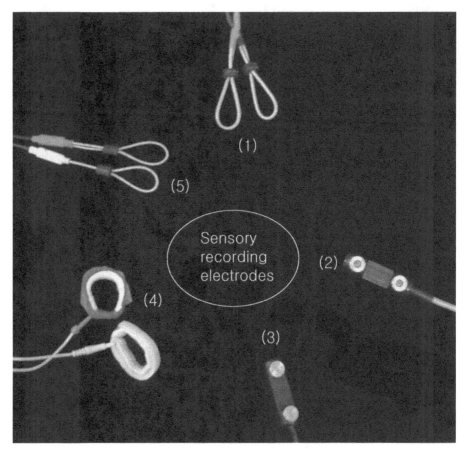

Figure 1-2. *Sensory recording electrodes.*

electrode. Recording and reference electrodes used for sensory responses usually are surface electrodes with a spring ring, disc, or bar (Figs. 1-1 and 1-2). Disc, bar, clip, and ring electrodes may be used interchangeably for recording and stimulating.

GROUND ELECTRODES

The ground electrode (Fig. 1-3) is a metal plate that provides a large surface area of contact with the patient. It serves as a reference zero potential and helps to reduce stimulus artifacts. The ground electrode usually is placed between the active electrode and the stimulator. It usually is larger than the recording and reference electrodes.

STIMULATING ELECTRODES

Surface stimulation electrodes usually are two metal electrodes or felt pad electrodes placed 1.5 to 3.0 cm apart (Fig. 1-4). The use of this stimulator is standard

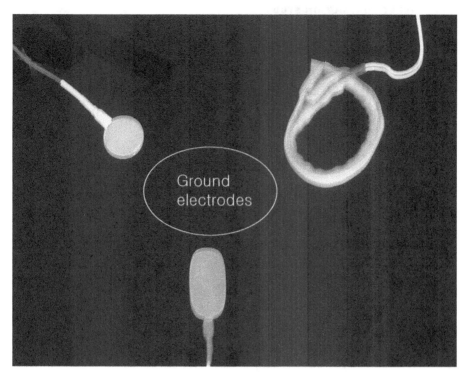

Figure 1-3. *Ground electrodes.*

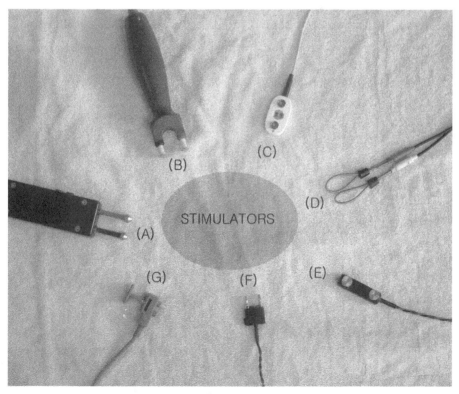

Figure 1-4. *Different types of stimulators.*

in conventional nerve conduction studies. However, the monopolar needle electrode also can be used for nerve stimulation. Its use has certain advantages: (a) a smaller stimulus intensity is required, (b) the nerve can be stimulated more selectively than with a surface stimulating electrode, and (c) nerves that lie anatomically deep can be stimulated (e.g., the spinal nerve roots or sciatic nerve in the sciatic notch).

Techniques: General Considerations

A few general rules make nerve conduction velocity studies easy to perform and greatly reduce the number of examiner errors. Ensure that the following steps are taken:

1. Cleanse all recording, reference, ground, and stimulating electrodes after each use by washing with warm soapy water. Each electrode should then be dried completely.

2. Electrically test all electrodes for broken wires or defective contact points. If a defect is noted, repair or replace the electrode.

3. Use a thin film of electrode gel on each electrode to maximize conductivity.

4. Ensure that the electrode site on the patient's skin is clean and free of oil, grease, and soil. The site should be cleaned and abraded, as necessary, to reduce impedance at the electrode/skin interface.

5. Mark all recording and stimulating points clearly with visible ink.

6. Measure distances with a tape measure that is closely apposed to the skin and anatomic course of the nerve.

7. Position the cathode (negative pole) of the stimulating electrode toward the active (recording) electrode for most of the studies presented in this manual.

8. Ensure that the stimulus is adequate to evoke a motor or sensory response. In general, a stimulus is defined as any external agent, state, or change that is capable of influencing the activity of a cell, tissue, or organism. In clinical nerve conduction studies, an electric stimulus generally is applied to a nerve or muscle. The electric stimulus may be described in absolute terms or with respect to the evoked potential of the nerve or muscle. In absolute terms, the electric stimulus is defined by a duration (current pulse width) in milliseconds (ms), a waveform, and a strength or intensity measured in voltage or current (milliamperes). With respect to the evoked potential, the stimulus may be graded as subthreshold, threshold, submaximal, maximal, or

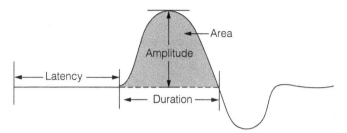

Figure 1-5. *CMAP parameters.*

supramaximal. The threshold stimulus is that stimulus sufficient to produce a detectable response. Stimuli less than the threshold stimulus are termed subthreshold. The maximal stimulus is the stimulus intensity after which a further increase in the stimulus intensity causes no increase in the amplitude of the evoked potential. Stimuli of intensities below this level but above threshold are submaximal. Stimuli of intensities greater than the maximal stimulus are termed supramaximal. Ordinarily, supramaximal stimuli are used for nerve conduction studies. By convention, an electric stimulus of about 20% greater voltage/current than required for the maximal stimulus should be used for supramaximal stimulation. The frequency, the number, and the duration of a series of stimuli should be specified on the reporting form.

9. Latency time (ms) for motor responses is measured from the shock artifact to the initial negative deflection (upward) of the response from the isoelectric baseline of the video display apparatus (Fig. 1-5).

With the motor nerve conduction velocity (NCV) technique, the reference and ground electrodes are placed over electrically inactive areas (Fig. 1-6). The active electrode is placed over the abductor pollicis brevis. The median nerve is stimulated supramaximally with bipolar surface electrodes distally at the wrist and proximally at the cubital fossa. The latencies from stimulus artifact to the initial negative deflection of the M response (T_A and T_B) are noted. The distance between the two sites of stimulation (D) is measured. The NCV in meters per second is calculated by dividing D by $T_A - T_B$.

10. Latency time (ms) for sensory responses is measured from the shock artifact to the peak of the negative phase or the initial positive dip of the sensory response (Fig. 1-7).

11. The amplitude in millivolts (mV) of the motor response is measured from the isoelectric baseline to the peak of the negative phase of the motor response.

12. The amplitude in microvolts (μV) of the sensory response is usually measured from the baseline to the negative peak or from the negative peak to the positive peak (peak-to-peak) of the sensory response.

13. The duration (ms) of the motor and sensory responses is measured from the initial deflection of the negative phase of the response from the isoelectric baseline to the return of the positive phase of the response to the isoelectric baseline

14. Conduction velocity (m per s) of a nerve is calculated by measuring the distance (mm) between two stimulation sites and dividing by the difference in latency (ms) from the more proximal stimulus and the latency (ms) of the distal stimulus. The equation is as follows.

$$conduction\ velocity\ (m/s) =$$
$$distance\ (mm)/proximal\ latency\ (ms) - distal\ latency\ (ms)$$

In the orthodromic technique, stimulating ring electrodes are placed on the digit with the negative (cathode) electrode placed proximally. Recording electrodes are placed over the median nerve at a standard distance from the stimulating electrodes. The latency (L) from the stimulus artifact to the initial point of the first negative deflection of the evoked nerve action potential is recorded.

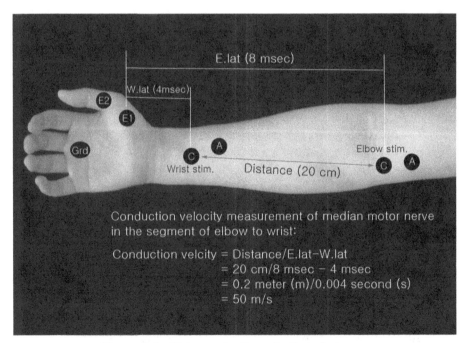

Figure 1-6. *Motor conduction velocity technique.*

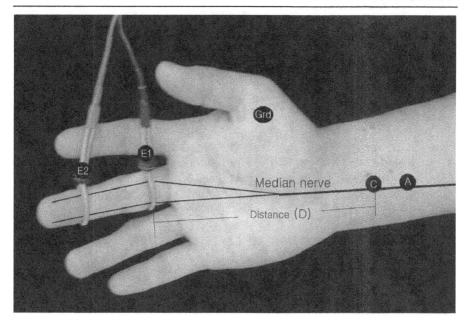

A

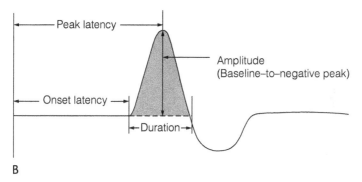

B

Figure 1-7. A: *Antidromic sensory conduction studies of the median nerve.*
B: *Sensory nerve action potential parameters recorded from antidromic*
median nerve conduction studies.

 Technical Procedures

The technical procedures for testing each motor and sensory peripheral nerve
presented in this manual are divided into five parts:

1. electromyograph instrument settings

2. patient position

3. electrode placement

4. electrostimulation

5. technical comments and illustrations.

The upper extremity nerves are presented first. The motor component of the nerve is described, followed by a description of the sensory component of the same nerve. The lower extremity nerves comprise the second half of the technique section and they are presented in the same format as those nerves in the upper extremity. Illustrations showing appropriate electrode placement, anatomic landmarks, and stimulation sites accompany each test description.

ELECTROMYOGRAPH INSTRUMENT SETTING

Filters: The filter settings for each technical procedure allow adequate instrument response to record the motor and sensory potentials being studied. The filter settings are 2 to 10,000 Hz for the motor potentials and 20 to 2,000 Hz for the sensory potentials.

Sweep Speeds: The sweep speeds for each technical procedure allow for display of the motor and sensory potential waveform. The sweep speed settings are 2 to 5 ms for the motor potentials and 1 to 2 ms for the sensory potentials per horizontal division on the video display apparatus.

Sensitivity: Sensitivity or gain settings for each technical procedure are general guidelines for recording the motor and sensory potentials. Increasing or decreasing the sensitivity settings may be necessary to accommodate very low or very high amplitude motor or sensory responses. Sensory sensitivity begins at 5 to 10 μV, whereas motor sensitivity is 1,000 to 5,000 μV per vertical division on the video display apparatus.

These are general guidelines and should serve as starting points for basic evaluation procedures. These settings should be modified to meet unusual or difficult evaluation settings.

PATIENT POSITION

The recommended patient position provides a comfortable, resting position for the patient. It also allows the examiner easy access to the extremity and nerve segment being studied.

ELECTRODE PLACEMENT

The active (recording) electrode is placed over the muscle or nerve segment being studied. The reference electrode for motor responses is positioned off and distal to the muscle being studied on a nearby bone or tendon. The reference electrode for sensory responses is placed distal to and on the nerve segment being studied. The ground electrode for the motor and the sensory responses is placed on a bony prominence between the stimulating and active (recording) electrodes.

ELECTROSTIMULATION

Percutaneous electrostimulation is performed with surface electrodes at appropriate anatomic locations along the course of the nerve segment being studied. For all techniques presented in this manual, the cathode (negative pole) of the stimulating electrode is positioned toward the active (recording) electrode. Stimulation sites are designated as S1, S2, etc., to identify the location and sequence of stimulation.

TECHNICAL COMMENTS AND ILLUSTRATIONS

Information considered useful for conducting an adequate and efficient evaluation is provided for each nerve. Cautions, special concerns, and recommendations for using the technical procedures also are included.

Medical illustrations showing electrode placement, stimulation sites, pertinent anatomic structures, and surface anatomy accompany each technical description.

Troubleshooting

When performing nerve conduction velocity studies, sometimes one cannot obtain a response. Because such nonresponse can result from many causes, a careful step-by-step analysis of the nerve stimulation technique is necessary.

MOTOR NERVE STIMULATION BUT NO RESPONSE IS SEEN

1. Check to be sure the stimulator is delivering an impulse. Most patients will feel the stimulus, but you can check it with your finger while turning up the voltage. If no stimulus is being delivered, then check the switches to see if they are set properly; remove the stimulator wires from their sockets and reinsert them properly. Next, check the stimulator wires for a defect, first visually and then electrically with an ohmmeter to determine whether the wire has electrical continuity. If, after following these steps, you find nothing amiss, then the problem lies within the stimulator. It must be tested by an electronics specialist.

2. If the stimulator is found to be working, then check the anatomical location of the stimulation electrodes. Occasionally, a beginner places the electrodes in the wrong area or over the wrong nerve.

3. If the stimulating electrodes are in the proper position, then check the amount of gel under the anode and cathode. Too much gel or sweating will create an anode-cathode bridge and will render nerve stimulation impossible. Little or no gel will deliver a submaximal stimulus strength.

4. If the stimulating electrodes are in the proper position, then stimulate. If there still is no response, increase the current pulse width of the stimulus slowly. This procedure often is necessary in extremely obese people or in those with edema or severe nerve disease.

MUSCLE CONTRACTION BUT NO EVOKED RESPONSE

1. Check the switch controlling the input in the preamplifier to be sure it is in the "on" position.

2. Confirm that the recording electrodes are over the motor-point area of the muscle being studied.

3. Remove excessive gel that can cause a bridge between the active and reference electrodes. This gel bridge will result in either a very small or no response. Add gel wherever it is insufficient under the recording electrodes. (Insufficient gel can have the same effect as too much gel.)

4. Check the recording electrodes and connecting wires with an ohmmeter to ensure electrical continuity.

5. On a multichannel electromyography (EMG) machine, if you still get no response, check the connections between the preamplifier and amplifier to ensure proper channel connections.

6. Check the ground lead. When the ground is not in contact with the patient, the trace on the video display apparatus will be off the screen.

7. Ensure that the display screen sweep speed is such that the expected response is on the screen.

8. Set the video display screen sweep speed so that the expected response is on the screen. (Try using a slower sweep speed, 5 or 10 ms per division, to see if the response is off the screen.)

9. In the event the evoked response is of low amplitude, increase the sensitivity by decreasing the gain on the amplifier to display the evoked response trace adequately on the video display apparatus.

STIMULUS ARTIFACT

If the record shows a large stimulus artifact, look into these possibilities:

1. The ground is not functioning. Be sure the ground electrode gel is adequate. Ensure that the ground is in contact with the patient. Be sure the ground electrode is located between the stimulating and recording electrodes. Test the electrode wire with an ohmmeter to ensure its electrical continuity.

2. A recording electrode is defective. Again, be sure the electrode gel is adequate, and the electrode and wire are checked with an ohmmeter for a defect. Defective electrodes should be repaired or replaced.

3. Check the stimulating electrodes to ensure there is no electrode gel bridge between the anode and cathode electrodes.

4. Make sure recording and stimulating electrode connection cables are not crossed and touching.

ABNORMAL RECORDED POTENTIAL

If the recorded potential voltage is abnormal, follow these steps:

1. Move the stimulating electrodes in small increments until the best response is obtained. Be sure the stimulus strength is supramaximal (submaximal stimulus may appear to give a decremental type of response, especially if the stimulator is not directly over the nerve).

2. Check the recording electrodes to ensure they are over the appropriate muscle and that the amount of electrode gel is adequate.

INITIAL POSITIVE DEFLECTION IN CMAP

If the evoked response seen on the display screen has an initial positive deflection, do the following, except for the posterior tibial nerve, where recording from the abductor hallucis usually results in an initial positive deflection.

1. Move the active recording electrode until it is over the motor point of the muscle.

2. Make sure the appropriate nerve is being stimulated and there is no volume conduction (crossover) to another, faster-conducting nerve (which can be checked by stimulating that other nerve).

3. Consider whether a crossover is present that would stimulate more remote muscles sooner than the one being tested.

4. Check for reverse electrode connections to preamplifier input jacks.

 Temperature Effects on Nerve Conduction Velocities and Latencies

Temperature can have the following effects on nerve conduction studies (Table 1-1).

1. Distal extremities are constantly exposed to environmental temperature changes.

TABLE 1-1.   Temperature effects on nerve conduction studies

	Sensory		Motor	
	Focal	*Diffuse*	*Focal*	*Diffuse*
Amplitude	↑	↑/NC	↑	↑/NC
Duration	↑	↑	↑	↑
Conduction velocity	NC	↓	NC	↓

NC, no change; ↓, decrease; ↑, increase.

2. There is a wide range of individual variation in response to environmental temperature changes.

3. The elderly have reduced adequate response to cold exposure. They have lower tissue temperatures than young adults when exposed to the same environmental temperature.

4. Patients with impaired circulation may have reduced tissue temperature and additional reduced NCV

5. Hemiplegic patients may have a lower skin temperature and motor NCV on the affected side compared with the unaffected side.

6. Borderline abnormal distal latency (DL) and NCV in patients with cool extremities may lead to erroneous diagnosis, such as peripheral neuropathy or entrapment neuropathy.

7. The ideal skin temperatures for performing EMG are as follows: upper extremity, 34°C; lower extremity, 32°C.

8. There are focal or diffuse cooling effects on nerve conduction studies.

CORRELATION OF SKIN TEMPERATURE AND NCV

1. Correlation of Skin Temperature and NCV is practical, painless, and quick.

2. Because skin temperature varies among sites in the parts of the extremities, a specific location for temperature measurement for each nerve has to be determined to standardize temperature correction to NCV

TEMPERATURE AND NCV CORRELATION FACTORS

Temperature and NCV correlation factors vary for the same type of peripheral nerve in the literature. This variation is partially due to different tissue temperature sites, depth of thermester needle, wider range to cooling, and species variation.

Suggested NCV correlation factors:

Use skin temperature measurements (range, 26°C to 32°C) to improve the accuracy of NCV studies:

Nerve	NCV (m per s per 1°C) skin	Skin temperature recording
Tibial motor	1.1	15 cm above medial malleous
Sural sensory	1.7	15 cm above medial malleous
Peroneal motor	2.0	15 cm above lateral malleous
Median motor	1.5	Distal groove volar midwrist
Median sensory	1.4	Distal groove volar midwrist
Ulnar motor	2.1	Distal groove volar midwrist
Ulnar sensory	1.6	Distal groove volar midwrist

Nerve	DL (ms)	Skin temperature recording
Median motor	−0.2	Distal groove volar midwrist
Median sensory	−0.2	Distal groove volar midwrist
Ulnar motor	−0.2	Distal groove volar midwrist
Ulnar sensory	−0.2	Distal groove volar midwrist

Equations

tibial motor NCV corrected = 1.1(skin temperature, 32°C) NCV (m per s).
sural NCV corrected = 1.7(skin temperature, 32°C) NCV (m per s).
peroneal NCV corrected = 2.0(skin temperature, 32°C) NCV (m per s).
median motor or sensory NCV or DL corrected
  $= CF(T_{st} - T_m) +$ obtained NCV or DL,
    where $T_{st} = 33°C$ for wrist, T_m is the measured skin temperature,
    and CF is the correction factor of the tested nerve.
ulnar motor or sensory NCV or DL corrected
  $= CF(T_{st} - T_m) +$ obtained NCV or DL,
    where $T_{st} = 33°C$ for wrist, T_m is the measured skin temperature,
    and CF is the correction factor of the tested nerve.

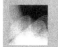 *Other Variability in Nerve Conduction Velocities and Common Sources of Error*

1. Sensory and motor conduction velocities are slower in the legs than in the arms, with differences ranging from 7 to 10 m per s.

2. Longer nerves conduct slower than shorter nerves.

3. Conduction velocities are faster in the proximal than in the distal nerve segments.

4. Age affects conduction velocities as follows:
   a. full-term infants: about half the adult values
   b. adult range obtained by age 3 to 5 years

    c. conduction velocities begin to decline at about age 40 years, but the decrease is less than 10 m per s by the 80th year.

COMMON SOURCES OF ERROR

1. Spread of stimulation current to adjacent nerves must be avoided or you will elicit unintended potentials. This can be a particular problem with peroneal and tibial nerves at the knee and the median and ulnar nerves at or above the elbow.

2. You must use supramaximal nerve stimulation or else erroneously prolonged latencies with small amplitudes will be recorded.

3. Excessive shock intensity can cause an unusually short latency by enlarging the electrical field and depolarizing the nerve segment away from the stimulating cathode.

4. Measuring the nerve surface length commonly overestimates or underestimates the conduction distance. Errors of measurement are amplified as the nerve segment shortens. Minimally, a 10-cm segment should be used.

5. Poorly defined takeoff points will result in errors in reading the beginning of the evoked response.

6. Some anomalies are as follows:
    a. Martin-Gruber anastomosis: 15% to 20% of people have an anomalous communication from the median to the ulnar nerve at the forearm.
    b. accessory deep peroneal nerve (20% to 28% of people): the anomalous branch of the superficial peroneal nerve supplies the lateral half of the extensor digitorum brevis

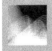 *Abbreviations*

E1, active recording electrode (old term, grid 1 = G1); E2, reference recording electrode (grid 2 = G2); CMAP, compound muscle action potential; NCV, nerve conduction velocity; mV, millivolt; μV, microvolt; ms, millisecond; m per s, meter per second; SSIS, short-segment incremental stimulation; EMG, electromyography; DL, distal latency.

 References

Campbell WW, Ward LC, Swift RR: Nerve conduction velocity varies inversely with height. *Muscle & Nerve* 1981;4:520–530.

Gassel MM: Source of error in motor nerve conduction studies. *Neurology* 1964;14:825–835.

Goodgold J, Moldaver J: Changes in electromyographic waveforms in relation to variation in type and position of electrode. *Arch Phys Med Rehabil* 1955;36:627–630.

Guld C, Rosenfalck A, Willison RG: Report of the committee on EMG instrumentation: Technical factors in recording electrical activity of muscle and nerve in man. *Electroencephalogr Clin Neurophysiol* 1970;28:399–413.

Gutmann L: Atypical deep peroneal neuropathy in presence of accessory deep peroneal nerve. *J Neurol Neurosurg Psychiatry* 1970;33:453–456.

Halar EM, Delisa JA, Brozovich FV: Nerve conduction velocity: Relationship of skin, subcutaneous, and intramuscular temperature. *Arch Phys Med Rehabil* 1980;61:199–203.

Halar EM, Delisa JA, Brozovich FV: Peroneal nerve conduction velocity: The importance of temperature correction. *Arch Phys Med Rehab* 1981;62:439–443.

Halar EM, Delisa JA, Soine TL: Nerve conduction studies in upper extremities: Skin temperature corrections. *Arch Phys Med Rehabil* 1983;64:412–416.

Kimura J: Principles and pitfalls of nerve conduction studies. *Ann Neurol* 1984;16:415–429.

Maynard FM, Stolov WC: Experimental error in determination of nerve conduction velocity. *Arch Phys Med Rehabil* 1972;53:362–372.

Rutkove SB: AAEM Minimonograph no. 14 The effects of temperature in neuromuscular electrophysiology. *Muscle & Nerve* 2001;24:867–882.

Simpson JA: Fact and fallacy in measurement of conduction velocity in motor nerve. *J Neurol Neurosurg Psychiatry* 1964;27:381–385.

CHAPTER 2

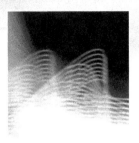

Cranial Nerves

 Facial Nerve

(Fig. 2-1)

Recording Electrode Placements (Fig. 2-2, Fig. 2-3)

E1 The surface recording electrode (E1) [10 millimeters (mm) in diameter] can be placed over the orbicularis oculi, nasalis, orbicularis oris, and frontalis muscles. When recording the motor response from any of the facial muscles, an initial positive deflection of compound muscle action potential (CMAP) is very common, but recording from the nasalis may yield the best result.

E2 The same type of E1 electrode is placed on the same muscle on the contralateral side of the face (E2).

Ground Place ground over the forehead or shoulder area.

Electromyography (EMG) Machine Settings

Filters: 2 Hz to 10 kHz

Sweep speed: 2 milliseconds (ms) per division (div)

Sensitivity: 500 microvolts (μV) to 1 millivolt (mV) per div

Current pulse duration: 0.2 ms

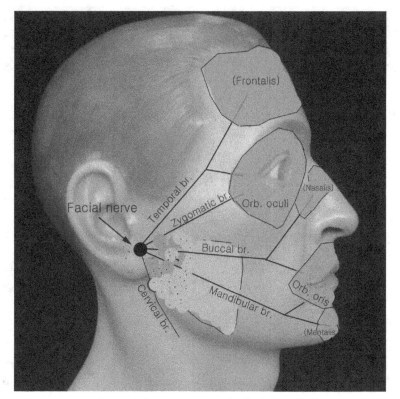

Figure 2-1. *Anatomy of the facial nerve.*

Stimulation of Facial Nerve (Fig. 2-5)

1. Preauricular stimulation: The stimulating cathode is placed over the anterior tragus in front of the ear. A volume-conducted response may occur with direct stimulation of the masseter muscle, but it can be minimized with the anode placed proximally to the cathode. We prefer stimulation at this site.

2. Postauricular stimulation (Fig. 2-5): The cathode is placed at the stylomastoid foramen, just behind and posterior to the lower ear and anterior to the mastoid process.

(Fig. 2-4) To supramaximally activate the normal facial nerve on pre- and postauricular stimulation, a moderate degree of current intensity is required. The stimulation is painful. We start the stimulation with 40 to 50 milliamperes (mA) with current pulse width 0.2 ms and monitor the CMAP amplitude changes with a gradual increase of intensity of 5 to 10 mA at a time until obtaining an optimal CMAP response. An intensity of 70 mA is usually enough for supramaximal stimulus in normal or diseased nerves. We also prefer the CMAP recording from three or four different facial muscles simultaneously using a multichannel recording system. For comparison of side-to-side differences of amplitude and latency, all technical factors for recordings from one side to another should be the same.

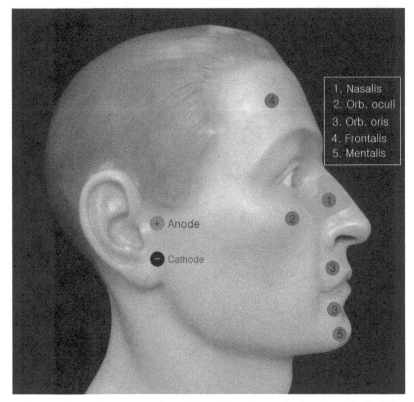

Figure 2-2. *Placements of recording electrodes and stimulator for facial nerve motor conduction.*

Reference Values

Kraft et al.[1]

Latency: 3.4 ± 0.8 ms

Amplitude: 2 to 4 mV

Waylonis et al.[2]

Age	Mean (ms)	Range (ms)
−1 month	10.1	6.4 to 12.0
1 month to 1 year	7.0	5.0 to 10.0
1 to 2 years (Y)	5.1	3.6 to 6.3
2 to 3 Y	3.9	3.8 to 4.5
3 to 4 Y	3.7	3.4 to 4.0
4 to 5 Y	4.1	3.5 to 5.0
5 to 7 Y	3.9	3.2 to 5.0
7 to 16 Y	4.0	3.0 to 5.0

Adult mean values: 3.4 ± 0.8 ms

[1] Kraft GH, Johnson EW: Proximal motor conduction and late response. AAEE workshop. Sept. 1986.
[2] Waylonis GW, Johnson EW: Facial nerve conduction delay. *Arch Phys Med Rehabil* 1964;45:539–547.

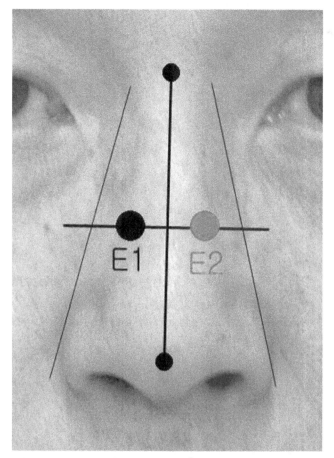

Figure 2-3. *Recording electrode placements in the nasalis muscle: E1 is active electrode and E2 is reference electrode.*

Coaxial recording from the orbicularis (Orb.) oris just superior to the corner of the mouth.

Korea University Medical Center **(KUMC)** (unpublished) $N = 60$

Muscle	Latency (ms)	Amplitude (mV)
Nasalis	3.8 ± 0.4 (2.4 to 4.8)	1.5 ± 0.6 (0.3 to 2.9)
Orb. oris	3.3 ± 0.4 (2.1 to 4.2)	1.9 ± 0.7 (0.5 to 3.5)
Orb. oculi	3.5 ± 0.5 (2.4 to 4.8)	1.9 ± 1.0 (0.3 to 5.6)
Frontalis	4.1 ± 0.6 (2.0 to 5.9)	0.8 ± 0.4 (0.03 to 2.1)

Surface electrode recordings.
Stimulation at the stylomastoid foramen.

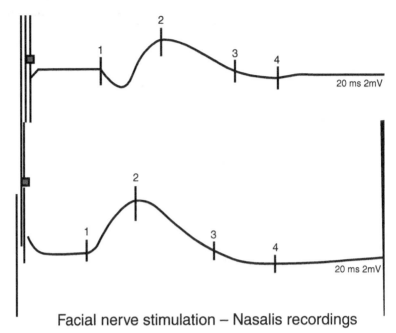

Facial nerve stimulation – Nasalis recordings

Figure 2-4. *CMAPs recorded from right and left nasalis muscles in facial nerve conduction studies. An initial positive deflection of CMAP in facial nerve conduction is common.*

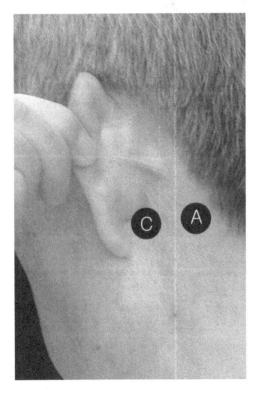

Figure 2-5. *A cathode (C) is placed at the styloidmastoid foramen for postauricular stimulation of the facial nerve. A, anode.*

Comments In the assessment of a proximal lesion, as in Bell's palsy, the latency of the direct response rarely is useful. Even with substantial axonal degeneration, the onset latency can be determined by the remaining axons to be normal or slightly increased. In contrast, the amplitude of the response provides useful information with regard to the prognosis by elucidating the degree of axonal loss. The CMAP amplitude varies substantially from one patient to the next. The comparison between sides in the same individual is more meaningful than the absolute value. An amplitude reduction up to one-half that of the CMAP on the normal side suggests distal degeneration. Serial determinations reveal progressive amplitude changes as an increasing number of axons degenerate. Distal excitability remains normal for a few days, even after complete separation of the nerve at a proximal site, but is lost by the end of the first week coincident with the onset of nerve degeneration. Prognosis is generally good if excitability remains normal during the first week after injury. With electrical shocks of very high intensity, stimulating current also may activate the masseter at its motor point. A volume-conducted potential from this muscle may erroneously suggest a favorable prognosis when in fact the facial nerve has already degenerated. The facial nerve on the face is divided into five branches: temporal, zygomatic, buccal, mandibular, and cervical. An isolated injury in one of these branches with facial trauma may occur but it is rare.

Trigeminal Nerve (Ophthalmic Nerve) Conduction Study

(Fig. 2-6)

Recording Electrode Placements

E1 The active recording electrode is placed on the supraorbital foramen.

E2 The reference electrode is placed medial to the E1 electrode.

Stimulation

The cathode of stimulator is placed at the upper lateral corner of the forehead.

Reference Values

Raffaele et al.[3] Subjects = 10   Age, 18 to 54 years

Latency (ms)   0.8 ± 0.1 (0.6 to 0.9) (to negative peak)

Amplitude (μV)   32.8 ± 2.8 (28 to 39) (peak-to-peak)

Conduction velocity (m/s)   59.1 ± 8.9 (43 to 73)

---

[3] Raffaele R, Emery P, Palmeri A, et al.: Sensory nerve conduction velocity of the trigeminal nerve. *Electromyogr Clin Neurophysiol* 1987;27:115–117.

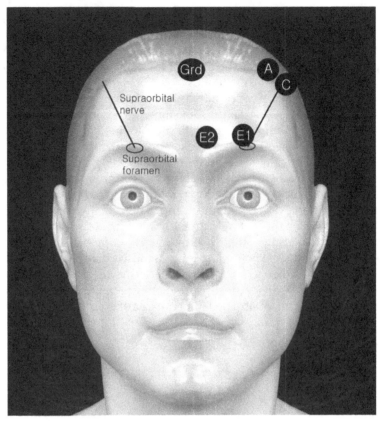

Figure 2-6. *Orthodromic trigeminal nerve conduction study. Grd, ground electrode.*

 Abbreviations

EMG, electromyography; ms, milliseconds; div, division; CMAP, compound muscle action potential; mA, milliamperes; mV, millivolts; Y, year; orb., orbicularis; μV, microvolts.

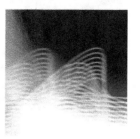

CHAPTER 3

Upper Extremity

Median Nerve

(Fig. 3-1)

MEDIAN NERVE MOTOR CONDUCTION

Median Nerve Motor Conduction Studies to the Abductor Pollicis Brevis (Fig. 3-2, Fig. 3-3)

Recording Electrode Placement

E1 The active recording electrode (E1) is placed on the most prominent eminence of the thenar area halfway between the midpoint of the wrist crease and the midpoint of the first metacarpophalangeal joint in the volar aspect. Thus, the E1 electrode is placed over the motor point of the abductor pollicis brevis (APB).

E2 The reference recording electrode (E2) is attached on the proximal phalanx of the thumb.

Stimulation

Wrist Stimulation is applied 8 (or 7) centimeters (cm) proximal to the E1 at the wrist, between the tendons of the flexor carpi radialis and palmaris longus.

Elbow The stimulator is positioned in the medial aspect of the antecubital space (crease), just lateral to the brachial artery.

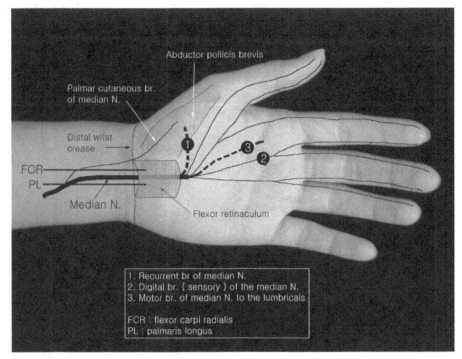

Figure 3-1. *Anatomy for median nerve conduction studies.*

Axilla This stimulation can be done between the biceps brachii and triceps muscles.

Erb's point (supraclavicular fossa) This stimulating point is located in the supraclavicular fossa, about 2 cm above the clavicle. Surface stimulation of the lower trunk, the origin of the median nerve to the APB, often is technically difficult because this trunk is located too deep.

Electromyography (EMG) Machine Settings

Filters: 2 hertz (Hz) to 10 kHz

Sweep speed: 2 milliseconds (ms) per division (div)

Sensitivity: 1 millivolt (mV) per div

Duration: 0.1 ms

Reference Values[1] $N = 47$

Distal latency (ms)	Conduction velocity (m/s)	Amplitude (mV)
3.7 ± 0.3	56.7 ± 3.8	13.2 ± 5.0

---

[1] Melvin JL, Harris DH, Johnson EW: Sensory and motor conduction velocities in the ulnar and median nerves. *Arch Phys Med Rehabil* 1966;47:511–519.

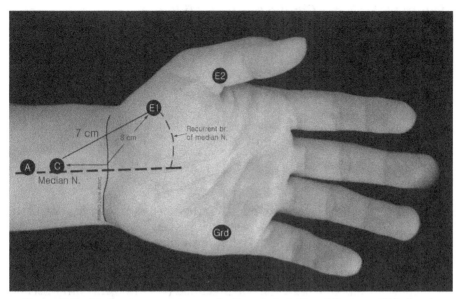

Figure 3-2. *Median nerve motor conduction study to the abductor pollicis brevis.*

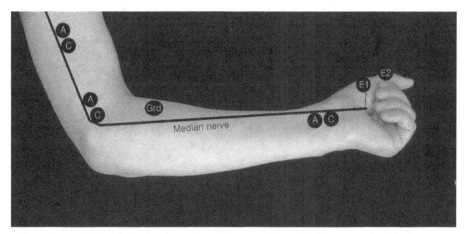

Figure 3-3. *Median nerve stimulations at the wrist, elbow, and midarm.*

Korea University Medical Center **(KUMC)** (unpublished) $N = 64$

Distal latency (ms)	Conduction velocity (m/s)	Amplitude (mV)
3.3 ± 0.4	57.4 ± 2.7	9.5 ± 2.7

Comments Before using any reference data, the author's recording instrumental parameters should be reviewed. High-intensity stimulation on the nerve may spread the currents to inadvertently stimulate the ulnar nerve at the wrist, elbow, or axilla.

Median Motor Nerve Conduction with Midpalm and Wrist Stimulation

Recording Electrode Placements

E1 and E2 electrodes: The APB muscle and proximal phalanx of the thumb.

Stimulation

Midpalm: Cathode is placed 3 to 4 cm distal to the distal wrist crease, along the distal margin of the carpal tunnel, with the anode proximal (Fig. 3-4).

Wrist: The stimulation is performed 8 cm proximal to the E1 electrode at the wrist.

Comments This method can determine whether there is any conduction block or delay of the median motor fibers as they pass the carpal tunnel area. The midpalm stimulations may show the following inadvertent effects: (a) activation of the ulnar nerve's deep branch; (b) direct stimulation of the motor point of the APB; (c) baseline distortion due to shock artifacts. Care must be taken so that the shapes of compound muscle action potentials (CMAPs) with both wrist and midpalm stimulations are similar.

Normal palm CMAP/wrist CMAP, <1.2 (120%)

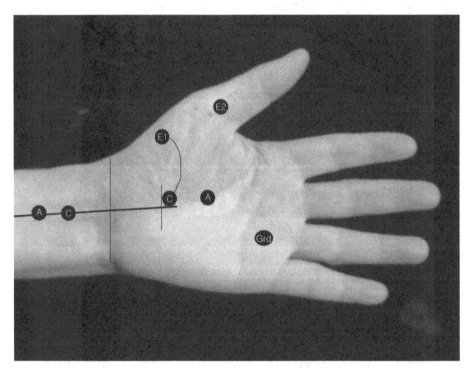

Figure 3-4. *Arrangements of cathode over anode for stimulation of the median nerve in the palm and wrist.*

Martin-Gruber Anastomosis (Median-to-Ulnar Anastomosis)

Recording Electrode Placements

E1 and E2 The surface recording electrodes are placed over the APB (E1) and its tendon (E2).

Stimulation Sites

Wrist and elbow, same as routine median motor nerve conduction studies.

Comments Anatomy: anastomosis is usually of the median nerve branching to ulnar nerve in the forearm (rarely ulnar to median).

a. Recognized easily in CTS (carpal tunnel syndrome) cases.

b. Unusually fast conduction velocity of the median motor nerve in the forearm.

c. In cases of severe CTS, wrist latency to the APB may be slower than the elbow latency to the APB with initial positivity of CMAP configuration with elbow stimulation.

d. In ulnar nerve motor NCS (nerve conduction study), ADM (abductor digiti minimi)-CMAP amplitude is larger with above elbow stimulation than with below elbow stimulated ADM-CMAP recordable with median nerve stimulation at the elbow.

e. One of two main anomalous innervations (Martin-Gruber, accessory peroneal nerve) is documented well in EDX (electrodiagnosis).

f. Martin-Gruber anastomosis occurs in 15% to 25% of patients.

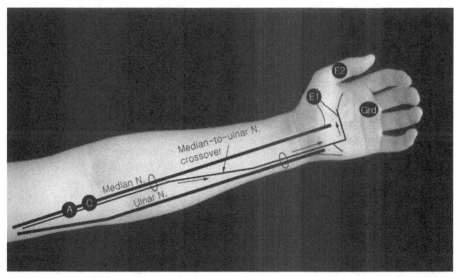

Figure 3-5. *Anatomy of Martin-Gruber anastomosis.*

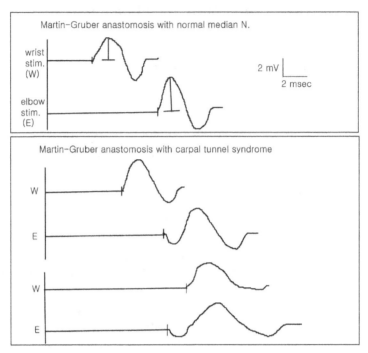

Figure 3-6. *Typical tracings of anomalies with median nerve conduction studies.*

Median and Ulnar Nerve Conduction to the Second Lumbrical and First Palmar Interosseous

Recording Electrode Placements

E1 The E1 is positioned in the midpoint between the second and third metacarpal bones in the palm side.

E2 The E2 is placed on the proximal phalanx of the second digit.

Stimulation

The stimulations of the median and ulnar nerves are performed at the wrist (Fig. 3-7).

Comments Supramaximal stimulation with surface electrode in the palm requires greater intensities than that of the wrist because the nerves are located more deeply under the thick palmar fascia and subcutaneous fat pad. This may lead to potential errors in measurement of motor conduction parameters (latency, amplitude, and morphology) because of inadvertent shock artifact or stimulus spread. However, this inching technique is highly sensitive to uncover the focal conduction abnormalities even mild sensory and/or motor fiber demyelination.

Reference Values

Abnormal: significant latency difference between median and ulnar nerves, ≥ 0.5 ms

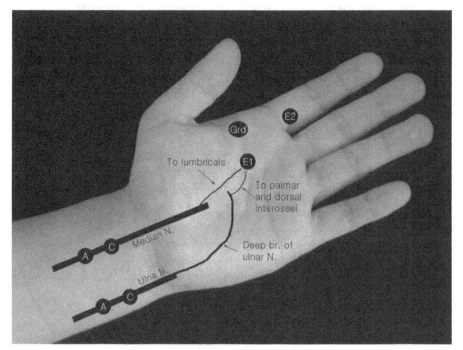

Figure 3-7. *Median and ulnar nerve conduction studies to the second lumbrical and first palmar interosseous.*

Anterior Interosseous Nerve Conduction to the Pronator Quadratus

Recording Electrode Placements

A standard concentric needle serving as E1 and E2 is inserted into the pronator quadratus about 2 cm proximal to the ulnar styloid process and between the space of the ulnar and radius bones in the dorsal aspect of the forearm (Fig. 3-8).

Mysiw and Colachis[2] used surface electrodes for recording.

Stimulation

The stimulus is applied just above the elbow between the medial epicondyle and biceps tendon, just lateral to the brachial artery.

Reference Values

Nakano et al.[3] $N = 84$

Latency: 5.1 ± 0.9 ms

No fixed distance was used.

---

[2] Mysiew WJ, Colachis SClll: Electrophysiologic study of the anterior interosseous nerve. *Am J Phys Med Rehabil* 1988;67:50–54.

[3] Nakano KK, Lundergan C, Okihiro MM: Anterior interosseous syndrome. *Arch Neurol* 1977;34:477–480.

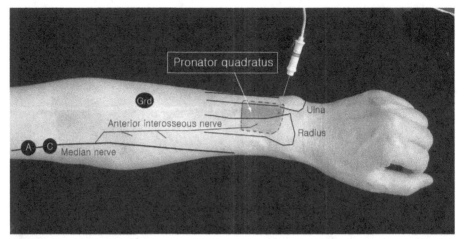

Figure 3-8. *Anterior interosseous nerve conduction study to the pronator quadratus with needle electrode recording. A concentric needle is inserted into the pronator quadratus through a space between the ulna and radius in neutral forearm position.*

Mysiw and Colachis[3] $N = 52$

Latency (ms)		Amplitude (mV)	
Right	Left	Right	Left
3.6 ± 0.4	3.5 ± 0.4	3.1 ± 0.8	3.1 ± 0.8

Distance: 17.5 to 28 cm (mean, 23 cm)

Anterior Interosseous Nerve Conduction Study to the Flexor Pollicis Longus

Recording Electrode Placements

E1 The E1 surface recording electrode is placed at the distal one-fourth of the volar forearm in the space between the brachioradialis and flexor carpi radialis tendons.

E2 The E2 surface reference electrode is attached to the radial styloid process at the wrist.

Stimulation

Stimulation can be applied proximally at the elbow, just medial to the brachial artery.

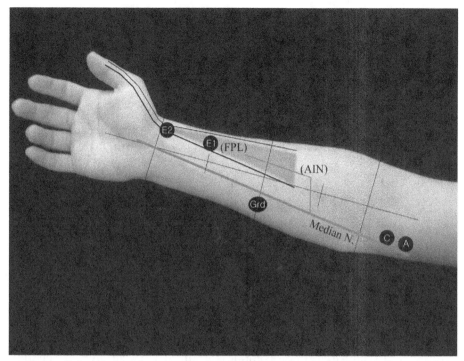

Figure 3-9. *Anterior interosseous nerve conduction to the flexor pollicis longus.*

Reference Values

Craft et al.[4] $N = 25$

Latency (ms)	Amplitude (mV)
2.6 ± 0.4 (1.8 to 3.6)	(5.6 ± 1.2) (3.8 to 7.5)

No fixed distance (9.1 to 10.2 cm) was used.

Felice[5] $N = 44$ Mean age = 38.3 years (range, 22 to 55)

Latency (ms)	Amplitude (mV)
3.6 ± 0.3	6.9 ± 1.1
(3.1 to 4.1)	(5.4 to 10.0)

---

[4] Craft S, Currier DP, Nelson RM: Motor conduction of the anterior intersseous nerve. *Phys Ther* 1977;57:1143–1145.
[5] Felice KJ: Acute anterior interosseous neuropathy in a patient with hereditary neuropathy with liability to pressure palsies: a clinical and electromyographic study. *Muscle & Nerve* 1995;18: 1329–1331.

Recording Electrodes: 1 cm × 2.5 cm strip surface electrode was used for both E1 and E2; E1 was placed transversely over the distal portion of the flexor pollicis longus, 7 to 10 cm proximal to the distal wrist crease; E2 was applied over the lateral aspect of the wrist; median nerve stimulation was applied 18 cm from E1 at the elbow.

Comments The shape of CMAPs often shows initial positivity and a rather complex form, likely due to a volume-conducted response from adjacent median nerve-innervated muscles. Care must be taken not to overstimulate the nerve at the elbow.

C-8 Root Stimulation with Monopolar Needle Electrode

Recording Electrode Placements (Fig. 3-10A)

The recording E1 and E2 are placed on either the abductor digiti minimi or the abductor pollicis brevis.

Stimulation (Fig. 3-10B)

To stimulate the C8 nerve root, a monopolar needle (Teflon coated) is placed between the C7 and T1 transverse processes, 1 to 2 cm lateral to the C7 spinous process, and a surface electrode as anode is arranged 2 to 3 cm lateral to the stimulating needle electrode. For measuring the conduction velocity, the distance between the C7 spinous process and the E1 recording electrode is measured.

Reference Values

Conduction velocity to

ADM: 68 ± 3 (m/s)

APB: 70 ± 2.7 (m/s)

Normal latency difference between the median and ulnar nerves, ≤1.7 ms.

Comments Comparison of the side-to-side latency difference may be useful to assess the proximal conduction abnormalities of the C8 root.

MEDIAN NERVE SENSORY CONDUCTION STUDY (FIG. 3-11)

Median Nerve Sensory Conduction to the Third-Digit—Antidromic Techniques[6]

Recording Electrode Placements (Fig. 3-12)

Antidromic median sensory nerve conduction studies can be performed with any of the four digits (digit I to IV). Using ring, clip, or bar electrodes, the sensory

---

[6] Johnson EW, Pease WS: *Practical Electromyography,* 3rd ed. Baltimore: Williams & Wilkins, 1997:154–156.

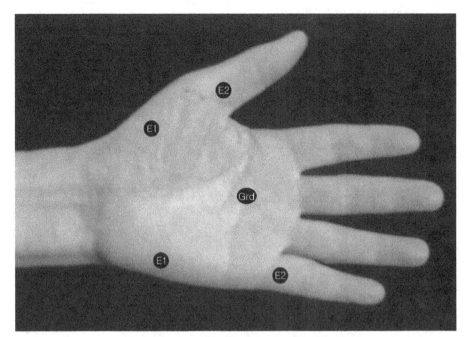

A

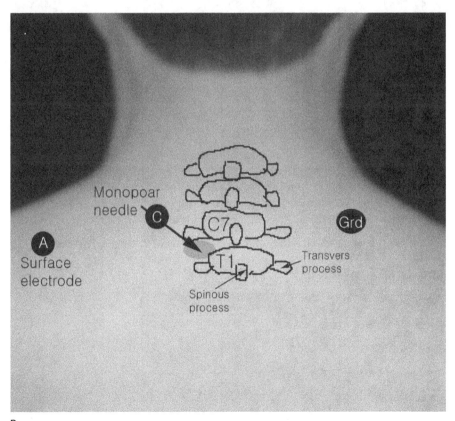

B

Figure 3-10. A: *CMAPs recording at the abductor pollicis brevis and abductor digiti minimi with C8 spinal root stimulation.* **B:** *C8 root stimulation.*

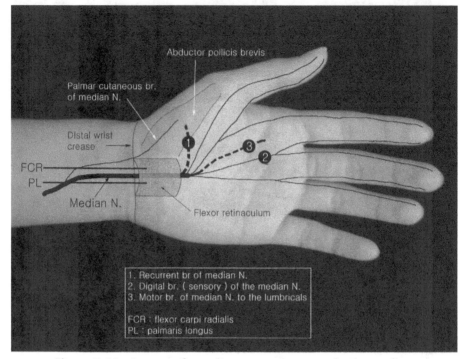

Figure 3-11. *Anatomy for median nerve sensory conduction studies.*

nerve action potentials can be recorded. When bar electrodes are used, the distance between the active and reference electrodes are fixed.

E1   In routine median sensory conduction, the E1 electrode is placed on the midpoint of either the second or third digit. We prefer the third digit recordings. The E1 placement requires some separation from the metacarpophalangeal joint to avoid volume-conducted muscle responses from the activated adjacent hand intrinsic muscles innervated by the median nerve.

E2   The E2 reference electrode is attached 4 cm distal to the E1 electrode.

EMG Machine Settings

Filters: 20 Hz to 2 kHz

Sweep speed: 1 to 2 ms per div

Sensitivity: 20 to 50 μV per div

Duration of pulse: 0.1 ms

Stimulation Sites

Wrist (Fig. 3-12) Stimulating cathode with anode proximal is placed 14 cm proximal to the E1 at the wrist between the tendons of the flexor carpi

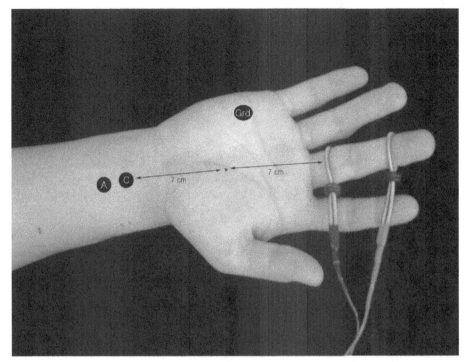

Figure 3-12. *Median nerve sensory conduction to the third digit.*

radialis and palmaris longus and ideally proximal to the distal wrist crease. Supramaximal stimulus is applied to the median nerve.

Midpalm The stimulation is applied 7 cm distal to the point of wrist stimulation at the midpalm, ideally distal to the carpal tunnel. On the midpalm stimulation, a short distance between the stimulating cathode and recording electrodes and higher stimulus intensities may evoke a distortion of sensory potentials due to shock artifacts. Rotation of the anode to the cathode in the palm may help to minimize the distortion.

Elbow Stimulate the median nerve just above the crease of the antecubital fossa and medial to the biceps tendon at the elbow.

Comments Measurement parameters include the onset and negative peak latencies and amplitude (baseline-to-negative peak) of compound sensory nerve action potential.

Normal values[7]		
Distal latency (ms) (peak)	Conduction velocity (m/s)	Amplitude (μV)
3.2 ± 0.2	56.9 ± 4.0	41.6 ± 25

[7] Johnson EW, Melvin JL: Sensory conduction studies of median and ulnar nerves. *Arch Phys Med Rehabil* 1967;48:25–30.

Korea University Medical Center **(KUMC)** (unpublished)
$N = 43$ Age 53.3 ± 9.1 (years old)

Stimulation site	Latency (ms) (to negative peak)	Amplitude (μV) (baseline to peak)
Wrist (14 cm)	3.3 ± 0.2 (2.9 to 3.8)	36.5 ± 8.3 (24 to 55)
Midpalm (7 cm)	1.8 ± 0.1 (1.6 to 2.0)	48.6 ± 10.9 (33 to 75)

Median and Ulnar Nerve Sensory Conduction Studies to the Fourth Digit

(Fig. 3-13)

Recording Electrode Placements

E1 and E2 Ring or bar electrodes are placed at the midpoint of the proximal phalanx in the fourth digit.

Stimulation The stimulation is performed 14 cm proximal to the E1 at the wrist for both median and ulnar sensory nerves.

Reference Values

Nerve	Latency to negative peak (ms)
Median	3.1 ± 0.2
Ulnar	3.0 ± 0.2

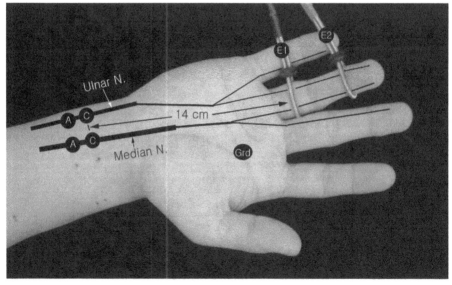

Figure 3-13. *Median and ulnar sensory nerve conduction studies to the fourth digit.*

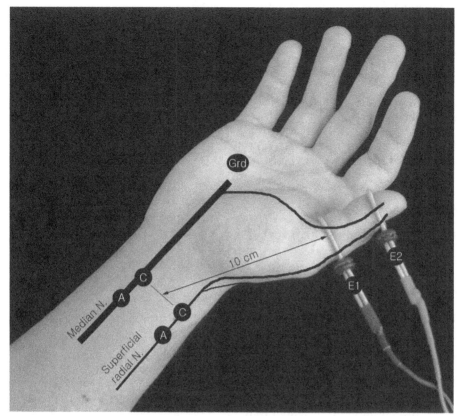

Figure 3-14. *Median and radial sensory nerve conduction studies to the thumb.*

Comments Comparison of latencies between the median and ulnar nerves is helpful to assess early or mild carpal tunnel syndrome. Significant latency difference between the median and ulnar nerves, ≥ 0.5 ms.

Median and Radial Sensory Conduction Studies to the Thumb

(Fig. 3-14)

Recording Electrode Placements

E1 and E2 Ring electrodes are placed around the thumb with an interelectrode distance of 4 cm.

Stimulation

The stimulations of the median and radial nerves are applied 10 cm proximal to the E1 electrode at the wrist.

Comments Comparison of latency difference for the median and superficial radial nerves is helpful to detect mild or early carpal tunnel syndrome.

[8] Johnson EW, Kukla RD, Wongsam PE: Sensory latencies to the ring finger: Normal values and relation to carpal tunnel syndrome. *Arch Phys Med Rehabil* 1981;62:206–208.

Reference Values[9]

Nerve	Latency to negative peak (ms)	Amplitude (μV)
Median	2.5 $\pm$ 0.2 (2.0 to 2.9)	30 $\pm$ 2.0
Radial	2.4 $\pm$ 0.2 (1.9 to 2.8)	12 $\pm$ 1.0

Normal negative peak latency difference between the median and superficial radial nerve, $\leq$0.5 ms

Median and Ulnar Sensory Nerve Conduction Studies Across the Wrist Over an 8-cm Segment

(Fig. 3-15)

Orthodromic Study: Median Nerve

E1 and E2 The recording surface bar electrode with E1 proximal is placed proximal to the wrist crease at the wrist between the tendons of the flexor carpi radialis and palmaris longus.

Orthodromic Study: Ulnar Nerve

E1 and E2 The same electrodes as above noted for the median nerve studies are placed near the flexor carpi ulnaris tendon at the wrist.

Stimulation

For stimulation of the median sensory (or mixed) nerve, the cathode is placed in the interspace between the second and third metacarpal bones near the palmar crease (longitudinal or proximal transverse creases). The ulnar nerve is stimulated in the interspace between the fourth and fifth metacarpal bones near the distal transverse palmar crease. The distance between the stimulation site and the recording E1 electrode is 8 cm.

Reference Values

Stevens[10]

1. Upper limit of normal for the median and ulnar mixed nerve peak latencies: $\leq$2.2 ms.

2. Significant latency difference between the median and ulnar nerves: >0.3 ms

Antidromic Short Segment Incremental Study—Inching Technique

(Fig. 3-16)

Recording Electrode Placements

E1 The recording ring electrode is placed over the proximal interphalangeal joint of the either third or second digit.

---

[9] Johnson EW, Sipski M, Lammertse T: median and radial sensory latencies to digit I: Normal values and usefulness in carpal tunnel syndrome. *Arch Phys Med Rehabil* 1987;68:140–141.

[10] Stevens JC: AAEM Minimonograph no. 26: The electrodiagnosis of carpal tunnel syndrome. *Muscle & Nerve* 1997;20:1477–1486.

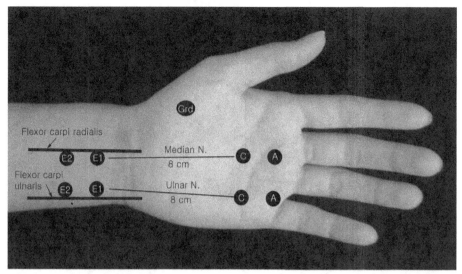

Figure 3-15. *Median and ulnar sensory nerve conduction studies across the wrist over an 8-cm segment.*

E2 The reference ring electrode is positioned around the distal interphalangeal joint of the same digit of the E1 recording electrode placed.

Stimulation

The stimulation is performed at 1-cm intervals distally or proximally from the distal wrist crease (0 point) along a 12-cm segment of the median nerve.

Comments

In cadaver dissection, the most narrow portion of the carpal tunnel is located approximately 2.5 cm distal to the distal wrist crease. This is probably the most frequent area of compression of the median nerve. This may be correlated with electrophysiologic findings by performing the inching technique to precisely locate the pathologic site.

Reference Values

Stimulation points (cm)	Latency change (ms)
−5 to −4	0.17 ± 0.08
−4 to −3	0.22 ± 0.10
−3 to −2	0.20 ± 0.09
−2 to −1	0.19 ± 0.08
−1 to 0	0.16 ± 0.08

−, distance distal to the distal wrist crease.

Normal range, ≤0.4 ms in 1-cm interval.

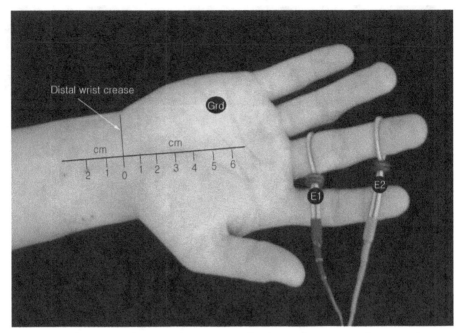

Figure 3-16. *Median nerve sensory conduction at 1-cm intervals across the wrist—inching technique.*

MEDIAN MIXED (MOTOR AND SENSORY) NERVE CONDUCTION STUDIES IN THE WRIST-TO-ELBOW SEGMENT

(Fig. 3-17)

Recording Electrode Placements

E1 For recording the compound nerve action potential, a plastic bar surface electrode can be used. The E1 surface electrode is positioned 4 cm proximal to the wrist crease between the tendons of the flexor carpi radialis and palmaris longus.

E2 It is placed distal to the E1 electrode.

Stimulation

The stimulation is performed at the elbow, just above the crease of antecubital fossa, lateral to the medial epicondyle and medial to the biceps tendon.

Reference Values[11]

Control $N = 16$ Age 21 to 63 years

---

[11] Pease WS, Lee HH, Johnson EW: Forearm median nerve conduction velocity in carpal tunnel syndrome. *Electromyogr. clin. Neurophysiol* 1990;30:299–302.

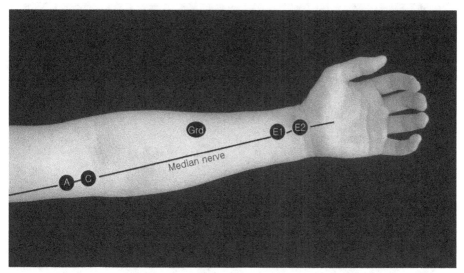

Figure 3-17. *Median mixed nerve conduction in the forearm segment.*

	Control	CTS patients
Direct forearm NCV (m/s)	54.4 ± 2.8	49.6 ± 5.0*
Standard forearm NCV (m/s)	54.5 ± 4.9	50.2 ± 6.0)*

* Significant difference ($p < 0.05$)

Comments Median motor nerve conduction studies were also performed with standard techniques. To obtain compound nerve action potential at the wrist, a relatively low-intensity stimulus [about 10 milliamperes (mA) with 0.1-ms duration] is required. Otherwise, the small responses are obscured by the volume-conducted compound muscle action potentials. A reduced conduction velocity has been reported in the patients with CTS.

PALMAR CUTANEOUS NERVE OF THE MEDIAN NERVE CONDUCTION STUDIES

(Fig. 3-18)

Orthodromic Technique—Chang et al.[12]

E1 The E1 active electrode is placed at the wrist, 10 cm from the stimulating electrode (C).

E2 The reference electrode is positioned 3 cm proximal to the E1 electrode.

Stimulation

The stimulation is performed at the midpoint of the thenar area.

---

[12] Chang CW, Lien IN: Comparison of sensory nerve conduction inthe palmar cutaneous branch and first digital branch of the median nerve: A new diagnostic method for carpaltunnel syndrome. *Muscle & Nerve* 1991;14:1173–1176.

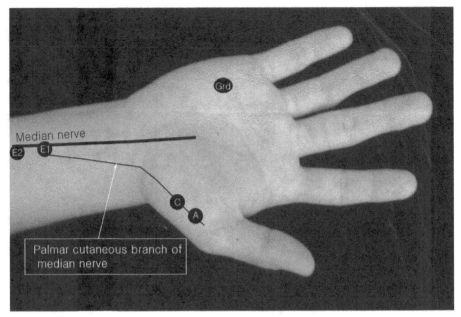

Figure 3-18. *Orthodromic conduction studies of the palmar cutaneous nerve of the median nerve.*

Antidromic Technique—Lum et al. [13]

Set-ups for the recording electrode placements and stimulation are just the reverse of the orthodromic method.

Reference Values

Chang et al.[12] $N = 40$ mean age $= 38.6$ years (22 to 60)

Latency to negative peak: 2.2 ± 0.2 ms (2.9 to 2.6)

Conduction velocity: 43.3 ± 3.5 (m/s) (39.2 to 52.2)

Lum et al.[12] $N = 50$

Latency: 2.6 ± 0.2 ms

Amplitude: 12 ± 4.6 μV

Comments Comparison of latency and conduction velocity differences between the palmar cutaneous nerve and first digital branch of the median nerve was useful to make the diagnosis of carpal tunnel syndrome (Chang et al.).[11]

---

[13] Lum PB, Kanakamedala R: Conduction of the palmar cutaneous branch of the median nerve. *Arch Phys Med Rehabil* 1986;67:805–806.

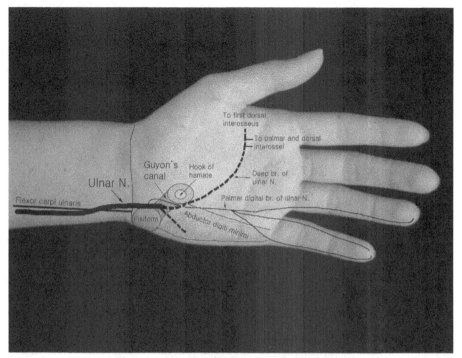

Figure 3-19. *Anatomy for the ulnar nerve conduction study.*

 Ulnar Nerve

(Fig. 3-19)

ULNAR MOTOR NERVE CONDUCTION STUDY TO ABDUCTOR DIGITI MINIMI

(Fig. 3-20)

Recording Electrode Placements

E1 The E1 active electrode is placed over the belly of the abductor digiti minimi.

E2 This reference electrode is attached on the proximal phalanx of the fifth digit.

Stimulation Sites

Wrist At 8-cm proximal to the E1 electrode, just lateral or medial to the flexor carpi radialis tendon at the wrist.

Elbow Approximately 3 to 4 cm distal to the medial epicondyle.

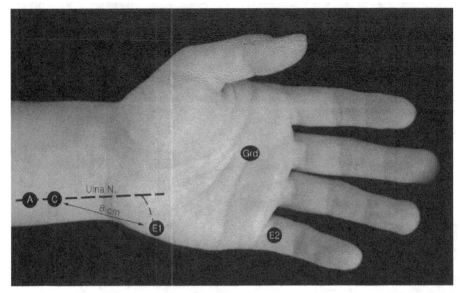

A

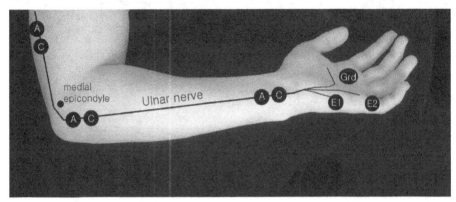

B

Figure 3-20. A: *Ulnar nerve motor conduction to the abductor digiti minimi.* **B:** *Stimulation sites for ulnar nerve motor conduction to the abductor digiti minimi.*

Mid-arm About 6 to 8 cm proximal to the medial epicondyle, between the biceps and medial head of the triceps.

Axilla

Elbow position during ulnar motor conduction A 70 to 135 degree of elbow flexion is recommended, but we prefer 90-degree flexion of the elbow for motor segmental studies.

Reference Values

Checkles et al.[14]

---

[14] Checkles NS, Russakov AD, Piero DL: Ulnar nerve conduction velocity: Effect of elbow position on measurement. *Arch Phys Med Rehabil* 1971;52:362–365.

$N = 31$ Subjects $= 18$ (20 to 58 years old)

Distal latency: 3.2 ± 0.5 ms

CMAP amplitude

Stimulation site	Amplitude (mV)	
	Elbow flexed 70 degrees	Elbow extended 180 degrees
Wrist	6.1 ± 1.9	6.1 ± 1.6
Below elbow	5.6 ± 2.0	5.3 ± 2.0
Above elbow	5.8 ± 1.8	5.4 ± 1.5

	Conduction velocity (m/s)	
	Wrist to below elbow	Across the elbow
Elbow flexed 70	61.8 ± 5.0 (53 to 73)	62.7 ± 5.5 (52 to 74)
Elbow fully extended	62.5 ± 4.5 (52 to 72)	49.9 ± 7.9 (34 to 66)

Kincaid et al.[15]

Subject $= 50$ (age range, 22 to 69 years old)

Segment	Conduction velocity (m/s)	
	Elbow flexed 135	Elbow fully extended
Below elbow to wrist	63.3 ± 5.2	65.7 ± 6.7
Above elbow to wrist	63.0 ± 4.7	59.0 ± 4.9
Axilla to wrist	62.6 ± 4.1	59.1 ± 4.2
Across the elbow	62.8 ± 7.1	50.3 ± 5.9
Axilla to above elbow	61.9 ± 6.0	60.9 ± 7.0

Buschbacher[16]

$N = 248$ Age: male, 44.7 ± 14.7 years; female, 40.8 ± 14.8 years

Measurement parameters	Mean $\pm$ SD	Normal limit
Distal latency (msec)	3.0 ± 0.3	3.6
Amplitude (μV)	11.6 ± 2.1	7.9
Nerve conduction velocity (m/s)		
Forearm segment	61 ± 5	51
Across elbow	61 ± 9	43
Above elbow	61 ± 7	47

Elbow position: 90 degrees flexed. Elbow stimulation: 4 cm below and 6 cm above.

Comments Checkles et al. described that a flexed elbow seems preferable for ulnar nerve conduction while it eliminates the elbow segment slowing in normal ulnar nerve found in the elbow extended position.

[15] Kincaid JC, Phillips ll LH, Daube JR: The evaluation of suspected ulnar neuropathy at the elbow. Normal conduction study values. *Arch Neurol* 1986;43:44–47.

[16] Buschbacher RM: Ulnar nerve motor conduction to the abductor digiti minimi. *Am J Phys Med Rehabil* 1999;78(Suppl 6): S9–S14.

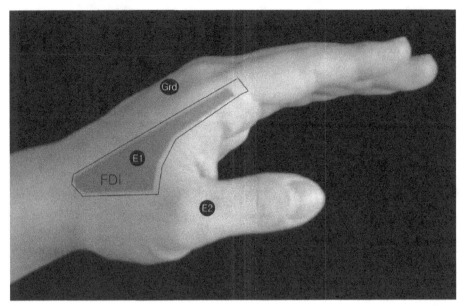

A

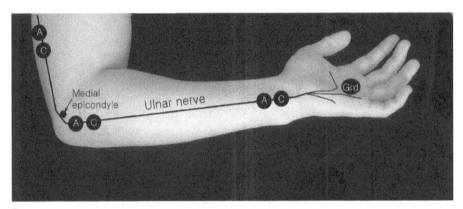

B

Figure 3-21. A: *Ulnar nerve motor conduction studies to the first dorsal interosseous.* **B:** *Stimulation sites for ulnar nerve motor conduction to the first dorsal interosseous.*

ULNAR NERVE MOTOR CONDUCTION TO THE FIRST DORSAL INTEROSSEOUS

(Fig. 3-21)

Recording Electrode Placements

E1 The E1 electrode is placed over the belly of the first dorsal interosseous.

E2 This reference electrode is attached on the dorsal aspect of the proximal phalanx of the thumb. The E2 placed over the index finger often shows an initial positivity in the CMAP.

Stimulation

The cathode is placed near the flexor carpi ulnaris tendon medially or laterally at the same stimulation point as that for routine ulnar motor nerve conduction to the abductor digiti minimi.

Reference Values

Olney et al.[17] $N = 373$ (subjects $= 188$)

Age (years)	Latency (ms) mean (range)		Amplitude (mV) mean (range)		N
	ADM	FDI	ADM	FDI	
<20	2.5 (2.2 to 2.9)	3.3 (2.7 to 2.9)	13 (11 to 16)	15 (8 to 23)	14
20 to 29	2.5 (2.0 to 3.0)	3.4 (2.6 to 4.1)	12 (5 to 20)	14 (8 to 22)	48
30 to 39	2.4 (1.8 to 3.2)	3.3 (2.5 to 3.4)	12 (6 to 21)	15 (6 to 24)	103
40 to 49	2.5 (2.0 to 3.0)	3.2 (2.3 to 4.2)	12 (6 to 19)	13 (6 to 22)	82
50 to 59	2.6 (2.0 to 3.4)	3.4 (2.6 to 4.4)	11 (7 to 17)	13 (6 to 20)	84
60 to 69	2.7 (2.2 to 3.1)	3.6 (3.0 to 4.1)	12 (6 to 15)	12 (7 to 20)	34
>70	2.7 (2.3 to 3.1)	3.6 (3.0 to 4.2)	10 (8 to 13)	12 (8 to 15)	8

Comments The distal motor latency to the first dorsal interosseous (FDI) should not exceed the distal motor latency to the contralateral first dorsal interosseous muscle by more than 1.3 ms; nor should this value exceed the distal motor latency to the ipsilateral abductor digiti minimi latency by more than 2 ms.

ULNAR MOTOR NERVE CONDUCTION STUDIES ACROSS THE ELBOW—SHORT-SEGMENT INCREMENTAL STUDY

(Fig. 3-22)

E1 and E2 placement The same as routine ulnar motor nerve conduction studies, the E1 and E2 are placed on the abductor digiti minimi or first dorsal interosseous.

Stimulation

Distal stimulation is applied 8 cm proximal to the E1 at the wrist, the same as for the routine ulnar nerve conduction studies. Segmental stimulation across the elbow is started 3 to 4 cm distal to the medial epicondyle and stimulation is proceeded/repeated proximally at 1- to 2-cm intervals) along the path of the ulnar nerve. We prefer the elbow to be flexed 90 degrees during the test.

Measurement Parameters: Changes of CMAP shape, amplitude, area, and latency, etc.

Reference Values

Kanakamedala[18]

---

[17] Olney RK, Wilbourn AJ: Ulnar nerve conduction study of the first dorsal interosseous muscle. *Arch Phys Med Rehabil* 1985;66:16–18.

[18] Kanakamedala RV, Simons DG, Porter RW, Zucker RS: Ulnar nerve entrapment at the elbow localized by short segment stimulation. *Arch Phys Med Rehabil* 1988;69:959–963.

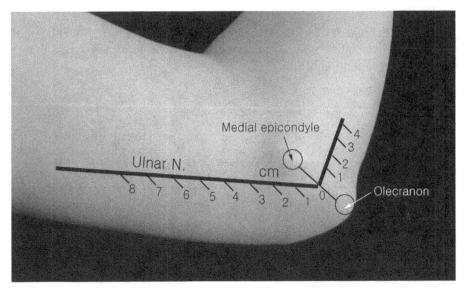

Figure 3-22. *Short-segment incremental stimulation of the ulnar nerve across the elbow.*

Ulnar motor nerve conduction studies across the elbow with 2-cm intervals.

Abnormal: right ($N = 12$), 0.63 ms (mean + 2SD = 0.43 + 0.2)

left ($N = 13$), 0.60 ms (mean + 2SD = 0.44 + 0.16)

Campbell[19]

Short-segment incremental studies (1-cm intervals) of the ulnar nerve at the elbow are performed with the elbow flexed 70 to 90 degrees. A latency change over a 1-cm segment more than 0.40 ms (mean + 2SD) is abnormal.

SHORT-SEGMENT INCREMENTAL STUDIES OF THE ULNAR NERVE AT THE WRIST[20]

(Fig. 3-23)

Recording Electrode Placements

The recording electrodes are placed over the belly of the FDI (E1) and the dorsal aspect of the proximal phalanx in the thumb (E2).

Stimulation Sites

The stimulation at 1-cm intervals is started 3 cm proximal to the distal wrist crease and continued distally ending 3 to 4 cm distal to the distal wrist crease. Higher-intensity currents may be required for the palm stimulations.

[19] Campbell WW, Pridgeon RM, Sahni KS: Short segment incremental studies in the evaluation of ulnar neuropathy at the elbow. *Muscle & Nerve* 1992;15:1050–1054.

[20] McIntosh KA, Preston DC, Logigian EL: Short-segment incremental studies to localize ulnar nerve entrapment at the wrist. *Arch Neurol* 1998;50:303–305.

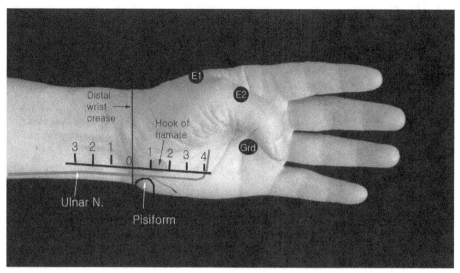

Figure 3-23. *Short-segment incremental stimulation of the ulnar nerve at the wrist with CMAP recording from the first dorsal interosseous.*

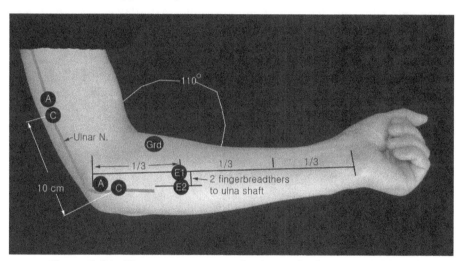

Figure 3-24. *Ulnar nerve motor conduction to the flexor carpi ulnaris.*

Comments The test is a valuable tool for the diagnosis and precise localization of ulnar nerve lesions at the wrist.

ULNAR NERVE MOTOR CONDUCTION TO THE FLEXOR CARPI ULNARIS

(Fig. 3-24)

Recording Electrode Placements

E1 The E1 surface electrode is placed over the motor point of the flexor carpi ulnaris, two fingerbreadths volar to the ulna at the junction of proximal and middle thirds of the forearm.

E2 The reference electrode is positioned over the shaft of the ulnar at the same distance posteriorly.

Stimulation

Below the elbow: Stimulation is performed 3 to 4 cm distal to the medial epicondyle.

Above the elbow: Stimulation is applied 6 to 7 cm proximal to the medial epicondyle so the total length of stimulating points across the elbow is 10 cm.

Reference Values[21]

	Latency (ms)		Conduction velocity (m/s)		Amplitude (mV)	
	AcE	AcE	BE	AE	BE	AE
Mean	2.6	4.2	1.6	63.0	5.2	5.2
SD	0.3	0.3	0.1	4.7	1.8	1.8
Range	2–3.5	3.4–5	1.4–1.9	52–71	2–9	2.1–9.5

BE, below elbow; AE, above elbow; AcE, across the elbow.

Comments Ulnar motor nerve conduction studies to the flexor carpi ulnaris may enhance more precise localization of ulnar neuropathies, especially when more distal recording sites are unavailable because of severe muscle atrophy.

SENSORY CONDUCTION

Ulnar Nerve Sensory Conduction to the Fifth Digit

(Fig. 3-25)

Antidromic Study

E1 A ring electrode is placed halfway on the proximal phalanx of the fifth digit.

E2 To maximize the sensory amplitude, a 4-cm separation from the E1 active recording electrode is preferred.

Stimulation Sites

Wrist Stimulation is performed 14 cm proximal to the E1 electrode, near the tendon of the flexor carpi ulnaris at the wrist.

Elbow Besides wrist stimulation, more proximal sites also can be stimulated below and above the elbow, the same sites for routine ulnar motor conduction studies with the same elbow positions.

Midpalm Stimulation is performed at the midpoint between the wrist stimulation and E1 recording sites in the midpalm area.

---

[21] Felsenthal G, Brockman PS, Mondell DL, et al.: Proximal forearm ulnar nerve techniques. *Arch Phys Med Rehabil* 1986;67:440–444.

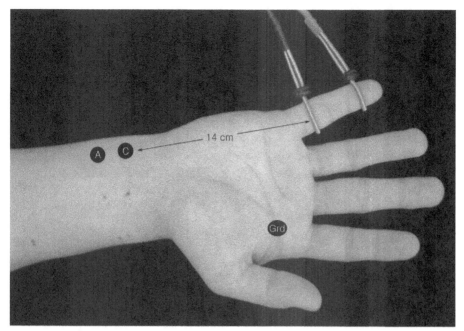

Figure 3-25. *Ulnar nerve antidromic sensory conduction to the fifth digit.*

Orthodromic study

Setups for orthodromic study, stimulation, and recording sites are exactly opposite those in the antidromic study.

Reference Values

Johnson et al.[22] $N = 120$

Latency to peak (ms)	Amplitude (μV)	Conduction velocity (m/s)
3.2 ± 0.3	15 to 50	57 ± 5.0

Latencies are the same for antidromic and orthodromic techniques.

Dorsal Cutaneous Nerve of the Ulnar Nerve

(Fig. 3-26)

Kim's Technique[23]

E1 and E2 A plastic bar mounted with the E1 and E2 electrodes is placed along the dorsum of the fifth metacarpal bone.

---

[22] Johnson EW, Melvin JL: Sensory conduction studies of median and ulnar nerves. *Arch Phys Med Rehabil* 1967;48:25–30.

[23] Kim DJ, Kalantri A, Guha S, Wainapel SF: Dorsal cutaneous nerve conduction: Diagnostic aid in ulnar neuropathy. *Arch Neurol* 1981;38:321–322.

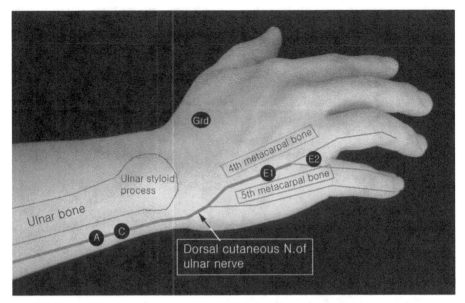

Figure 3-26. *Dorsal cutaneous nerve of ulnar nerve conduction study.*

Stimulation

Stimulation is applied 8 to 10 cm proximal to the ulnar styloid between the flexor carpi ulnaris and ulna where the nerve becomes superficial.

Reference Values

$N = 66$ Age, 21 to 71 years

Latency (peak) (ms)	Amplitude (peak-to-peak, μV)	Conduction velocity (m/s)
2.1 ± 0.3	24.2 ± 10.8	47.8 ± 3.8

Average distance for conduction studies, 11 to 12 cm.

Jabre's Technique[24]

E1 and E2 The bar electrode is positioned on the dorsum of the hand at the bottom of the V formed between the fourth and fifth metacarpal bones (this space can be palpated).

Stimulation

The stimulation site is the same as noted above, 8 cm proximal to the active recording electrode E1.

---

[24] Jabre JF: Ulnar nerve lesions at the wrist: New techniques for recording from the sensory dorsal branch of the ulnar nerve. *Neurology* 1980;30:873–876.

Reference Values

$N = 50$ in 30 subjects Age, 10 to 66 years

Latency (ms)	Amplitude (peak-to-peak, μV)	Conduction velocity (m/s)
2.0 ± 0.3	20 ± 6.0	$60 \pm 4.0\,(N = 16)$

Comments The sensory conduction is useful for localizing a lesion of the ulnar nerve segment proximal to a wrist lesion when the routine ulnar motor and sensory conduction studies are abnormal.

Radial Nerve

MOTOR NERVE CONDUCTION STUDIES TO THE EXTENSOR INDICIS

(Fig. 3-27)

Recording Electrode Placements

E1 A monopolar needle or surface recording electrode is placed 2 to 4 cm proximal to the ulnar styloid process on the dorsal aspect of the forearm, near the lateral edge of the ulnar bone.

E2 It is positioned distal to the E1 electrode, on the ulnar styloid process.

Stimulation Sites

Distal (forearm) A stimulating cathode is placed 4 to 6 cm proximal to the E1 electrode along the lateral edge of the ulna.

Elbow It is stimulated 5 to 6 cm proximal to the lateral epicondyle of humerus, between the biceps brachii and brachioradialis muscles.

Arm To test the upper arm segment of the radial nerve in the region of the spiral groove, the nerve is stimulated just posterior to the deltoid muscle insertion.

Erb's point To test the entire radial nerve distal to Erb's point, it is stimulated in the supraclavicular fossa (at the angle of the clavicle and posterior aspect of the sternocleidomastoid muscle).

Distance Measurement: Jebsen Technique

The distance is measured by using a tape between the above elbow and forearm sites. An obstetrical caliper is used for a straight line measurement from Erb's point to the above-elbow site. The arm is abducted 10 degrees, the elbow flexed 10 to 15 degrees, and the forearm pronated fully.

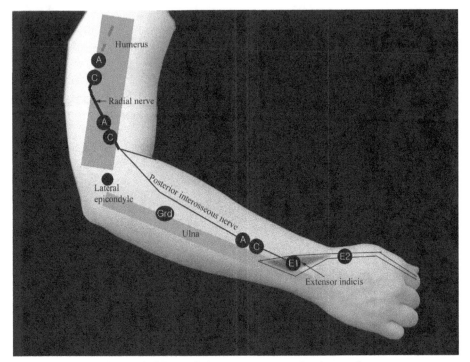

Figure 3-27. *Radial nerve motor conduction study.*

Reference Values

Jebsen[25] $N = 98$ (subject, 49) Mean age = 32.5 years (18 to 58)

Segment	Conduction velocity (m/s)
Forearm to above elbow	61.6 ± 5.9 (48 to 75)
Above elbow to Erb's point	72.0 ± 6.3 (56 to 93)

Needle recording was performed in the extensor indicis.

Trojaborg and Sindrup[26]

Segment	Conduction velocity (m/s)
Muscle to forearm	2.4 ± 0.5
Forearm to elbow	62.0 ± 5.1
Elbow to axilla	69.0 ± 5.6

Comments The CMAP recording with surface electrodes usually has an initial positive deflection of CMAP. Stimulation in the arm or axilla often is technically difficult. A standardization of distance measurement is also difficult.

[25] Jebsen RH: Motor conduction velocity in proximal and distal segment of the radial nerve. *Arch Phys Med Rehabil* 1966;47:597–602.

[26] Trojaborg W, Sindrup EH: Motor and sensory conduction in different segments of the radial nerve in normal subjects. *J Neurol Neurosurg Psychiatry* 1969;32:354–359.

RADIAL NERVE SENSORY CONDUCTION STUDIES: SUPERFICIAL RADIAL NERVE

Recording Sites:

Anatomic snuffbox area recording

(Fig. 3-28)

Recording electrode placements

E1 The surface electrode is placed in the anatomic snuffbox, which is bordered by the tendons of the extensor pollicis longus and brevis and the distal margin of the radius at the wrist.

E2 The E2 electrode is attached on the lateral side of the second metacarpal bone.

Stimulation

The superficial radial nerve courses along the lateral border of the radius with the radial artery in the volar aspect of the forearm. Stimulation is applied 10, 12, or 14 cm proximal to the E1 recording electrode with the cathode placed distally.

Reference Values[27]

Distance (cm)	Latency (ms) (mean ± 2SD)
10	2.3 ± 0.4
12	2.6 ± 0.4
14	2.9 ± 0.4

Sweep speed, 2 ms/div

Thumb recording
(Fig. 3-29)

E1 and E2 The ring electrodes are placed on the thumb: E1 is placed near the metacarpopharyngeal joint; E2 is placed on the distal interphalangeal joint.

Stimulation

The stimulating electrode is placed over the lateral side of the radius in the volar aspect of forearm near the radial artery, which can be palpated. Stimulation is applied 14, 16, and 18 cm from the E1 electrode.

Reference Values $N = 49$

Distance (cm)	Latency (ms) (mean ± 2SD)		Amplitude (μV)
	Onset	Peak	
14	2.8 ± 0.5	3.3 ± 0.6	12 ± 8 (7 to 19)
16	3.1 ± 0.5	3.6 ± 0.6	
18	3.5 ± 0.6	3.9 ± 0.6	

---

[27] Mackenzie K, DeLisa JA: Determining the distal sensory latency of the superficial radial nerve in normal adult subjects. *Arch Phys Med Rehabil* 1981;62:31–34.

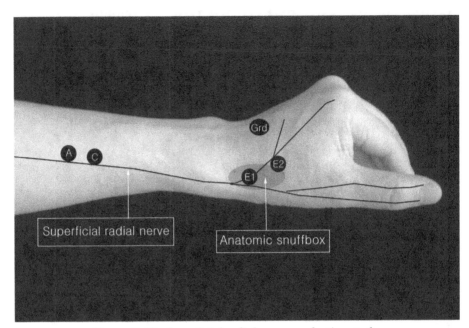

Figure 3-28. *Superficial radial nerve conduction study.*

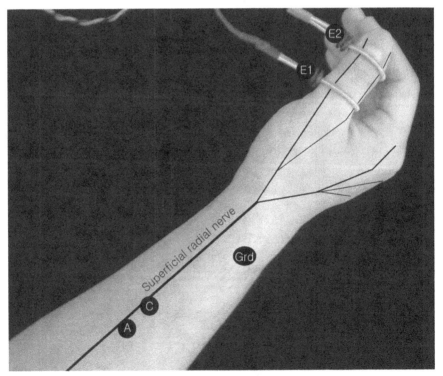

Figure 3-29. *Superficial radial nerve conduction study.*

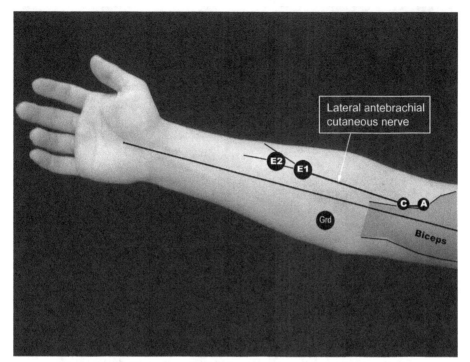

Figure 3-30. *Lateral antecubital cutaneous nerve conduction study.*

LATERAL ANTEBRACHIAL CUTANEOUS NERVE

(Fig. 3-30)

Recording Electrode Placements

E1 The stimulating point of the nerve is located over the crossing point between the lateral border of the biceps tendon and crease of the antecubital fossa. From this point, a line is drawn to the radial artery at the wrist. The E1 recording electrode is attached on the above noted line 12 cm distal to the stimulation point.

E2 The reference electrode is positioned 4 cm distal to the E1 electrode.

Stimulation

The stimulator is placed on the elbow crease and immediately lateral to the border of the biceps tendon at the elbow. The sensory nerve is superficial in this area.

Reference Values

Spindler et al.[28] $N = 60$ (subject, 30 adults)

[28] Spindler HA, Felsenthal G: Sensory conduction in the musculocutaneous nerve. *Arch Phys Med Rehabil* 1978;59:20–23.

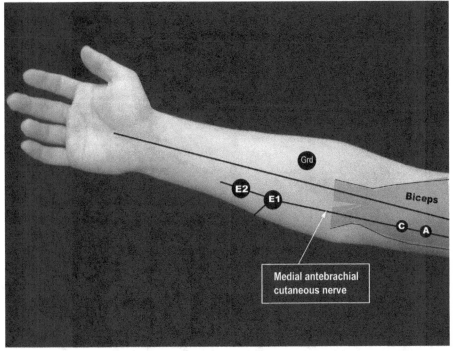

Figure 3-31. *Medial antebrachial cutaneous nerve conduction study.*

Latency (ms)		Amplitude (μV)	Conduction velocity (m/s)
Onset	Peak		
1.8 ± 0.1	2.3 ± 0.1	24 ± 7.2	65 ± 3.6
(1.6 to 2.1)	(2.2 to 2.6)	(12 to 50)	

Izzo et al.[29] *N* = 154 Mean age = 45.1 years (17 to 80)

Latency (peak) (ms)	Amplitude (μV)	Conduction velocity (m/s)
2.8 ± 0.2	18.9 ± 9.9	62.0 ± 4.0

Distance, 14 cm

MEDIAL ANTEBRACHIAL CUTANEOUS NERVE

(Fig. 3-31)

Recording Electrode Placements

E1 From the midpoint between the medial epicondyle and the biceps tendon, a line can be drawn to the ulnar side of the wrist just lateral to the flexor carpi

---

[29] Izzo KL, Aravabhumi S, Jafri A, et al.: Medial and lateral antebrachial cutaneous nerves: Standardization of technique, reliability and age effect on healthy subjects. *Arch Phys Med Rehabil* 1985;66:592–597.

ulnaris tendon. The E1 recording electrode is placed 8 to 10 cm distal to the above noted midpoint on the line drawn.

E2 The E2 reference electrode is attached 4 cm distal to the E1 active electrode.

Stimulation

The cathode is placed 2 to 4 cm extended proximally from the midpoint as it is described, over the medial aspect of the biceps muscle. For stimulation, care must be taken to use a low-intensity current, use a short duration of pulse, and apply light pressure to the cathode. Otherwise, the median and ulnar nerves that are located nearby can be easily coactivated.

Reference Values

Pribyl et al.[30] $N = 40$

Latency (peak) (ms)	Amplitude (μV)	Conduction velocity (m/s)
1.7 to 2.6 (mean, 2.1)	10 to 30 (mean, 20)	49.3 to 3.8

Distances for conduction study, 9 to 12 cm.

Izzo et al.[31] $N = 155$ Mean age = 45.1 years (17 to 80)

Latency (peak) (ms)	Amplitude (μV)	Conduction velocity (m/s)
2.7 ± 0.2	11.4 ± 5.2	63 ± 5

Distance, 14 cm

POSTERIOR ANTEBRACHIAL CUTANEOUS NERVE

(Fig. 3-32)

Recording Electrode Placements

E1 The E1 active recording electrode is positioned 12 cm distal along a line extending from the stimulating point to the middorsum of the wrist (midway between the ulnar and radial styloid processes).

E2 The reference E2 electrode is placed 3 cm distal to the E1 electrode.

Stimulation

The stimulating cathode is applied just above the lateral epicondyle, between the biceps brachii and the lateral head of the triceps muscle, closer to the latter. Stimulation can be given just above the lateral epicondyle, 0.5 to 2 cm away, and readjusted anteriorly or posteriorly in search for the optimal stimulation site.

[30] Pribyle R, You SB, Jantra P: Sensory nerve conduction velocity of the medial antebrachial cutaneous nerve. *Electromyogr Clin Neurophysiol* 1979;19:41–46.

[31] Izzo KL, Aravabhumi S, Jafri A, et al.: Medial and lateral antebrachial cutaneous nerves: Standardization of technique, reliability and age effect on healthy subjects. *Arch Phys Med Rehabil* 1985;66: 592–597.

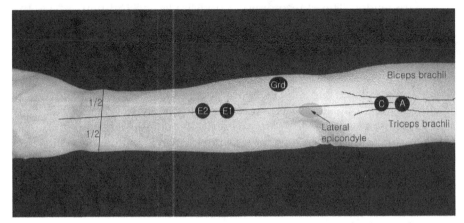

Figure 3-32. *Posterior antebrachial cutaneous nerve conduction study.*

Reference Values

Ma et al.[32] $N = 40$ (subject, 22) Age, 19 to 48 years

Latency (onset) (ms)	Amplitude (peak to peak) (μV)	Conduction velocity (m/s)
1.9 ± 0.3	8.6 ± 3.9	64 ± 7.4
(range, 1.5 to 2.4)	(range, 5 to 20)	

H Reflex of the Flexor Carpi Radialis

Jabre's Technique[33]

(Fig. 3-33A)

Recording Electrode Placements

E1 The E1 surface recording electrode is placed over the belly of the flexor carpi radialis, which is at about one-third of the line between the medial epicondyle and the radial styloid process.

E2 The reference electrode is attached lateral to the E1 over the brachioradialis muscle.

Stimulation

The cathode of bipolar surface electrodes is positioned just lateral to the medial epicondyle at the elbow with the anode distal.

---

[32] Ma DM, Liveson JA: *Laboratory reference for clinical neurophysiology.* Philadelphia: FA Davis. 1992: 72–75.

[33] Jabre JF: Surface recording of the H reflex of the flexor carpi radialis. *Muscle & Nerve* 1981;4:435–438.

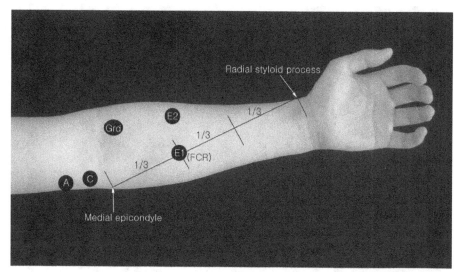

A

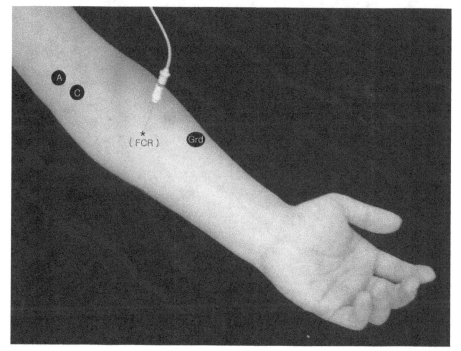

B

Figure 3-33. *A: Surface electrode recording of H reflex in the flexor carpi radialis.*
B: H reflex studies in the flexor carpi radialis with needle electrode recording.

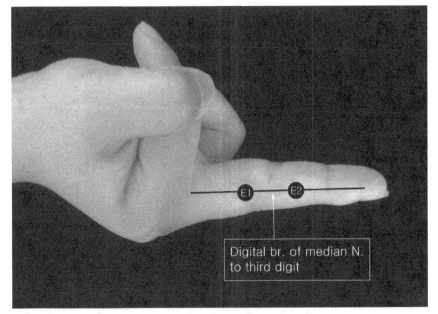

A

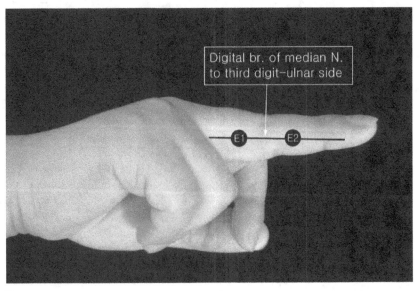

B

Figure 3-34. *A and B: Placements of recording electrodes for unilateral digital branch of the median nerve.*

EMG Machine Settings

Filters, 20 Hz to 10 kHz

Sweep speed, 5 ms/div

Sensitivity, 200 μV/div

Pulse duration, 0.5 to 1.0 ms

Stimulation frequency, <0.5 Hz

Reference Values

$N = 50$ (subjects, 30) Age, 15 to 56 years

Latency (ms)	Amplitude (mV)
15.9 ± 1.5	1.6 ± 0.4

Side-to-side difference, <1.0 ms

Unobtainable H reflex in normal individual, 10%

de Visser's Technique [34]

(Fig. 3-33B)

Recording Electrode Placement

E1 and E2 A standard concentric needle is placed over the muscle belly of the flexor carpi radialis, similar to Jabre's technique.

Stimulation Site and EMG Settings

Similar to Jabre's approach.

Reference Values

(B) Subject $= 52$ Mean age $= 50.8$ years (range, 20 to 85)

Latency (ms)	Side-to-side difference (ms)
16.8 ± 1.1	2.4 ± 0.38

Comments The response can be facilitated by minimal to moderate voluntary contraction of the wrist by the flexor carpi radialis. H reflexes can provide complementary information in identifying the lesion of the C6 and C7 nerve roots or brachial plexopathy.

Palmar Unilateral Digital Branch of Median and Ulnar Nerve Conduction Studies

(Fig. 3-34)

E1 and E2 The E1 and E2 surface recording electrodes mounted in a plastic bar are placed on one side of the finger with the E1 positioned at the midpoint of

---

[34] de Visser O, Schimsheimer RJ, Hart AAM: The H reflex of the flexor carpi radialis muscle: A study in controls and radiation-induced brachial plexus lesion. *J Neurol Neurosurg Psychiatry* 1984;47: 1098–1101.

the proximal phalanx with the E2 distal. An exactly identical bar electrode is attached on the opposite side of the finger at the same level. The fingers and digital nerves to be tested are as follows:

First digit, median and radial nerves

Second digit, median nerve

Third digit, median nerve

Fourth digit, median and ulnar nerves

Fifth digit, ulnar nerve

Stimulation

Stimulations for the median, ulnar, and radial nerves are performed as routine sensory conduction studies.

Comments Side-to-side comparison of amplitude and latency may be helpful for estimating an isolated digital nerve lesion, although a volume-conducted response from an intact digital branch on the opposite side cannot be avoided.

 Abbreviations

APB, abductor pollicis brevis; EMG, electromyography; cm, centimeter; Hz, hertz; ms, millisecond; div, division; mV, millivolt; CMAP, compound muscle action potential; μV, microvolt; mA, milliampere; FDI, first dorsal interosseus.

CHAPTER 4

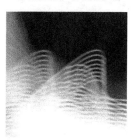

Lower Extremity

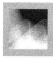
Common Peroneal Nerve

(Fig. 4-1, Fig. 4-2)

PERONEAL NERVE MOTOR CONDUCTION STUDY[1]

Recording Electrode Placements

E1 The E1 electrode is placed over the belly of the extensor digitorum brevis.

E2 The E2 electrode is positioned over the metatarsophalangeal joint of the little toe.

Stimulation

For routine peroneal motor conduction studies, stimulations are applied in three sites.

Ankle: Stimulation is applied 8 cm proximal to the E1, just lateral to the tibialis anterior tendon. At times, high intensities of current are required to stimulate the nerve because it is deep beneath the tendon, thick skin, or edema. Occasionally, the nerve is displaced more laterally so the stimulating cathode needs to move laterally to the nerve's close proximity.

---

[1] Jimenez J, Easton JK, Redford JB: Conduction studies of the anterior and posterior tibial nerves. *Arch Phys Med Rehabil* 1970;51:164–169.

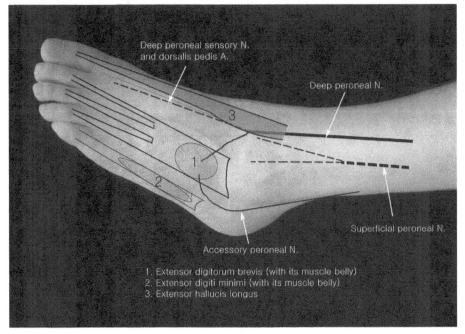

A

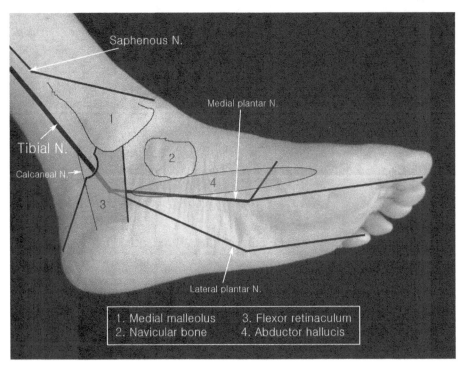

B

Figure 4-1. *A: Anatomy of the dorsum of the foot. B: Anatomy of the ankle-flexor retinaculum.*

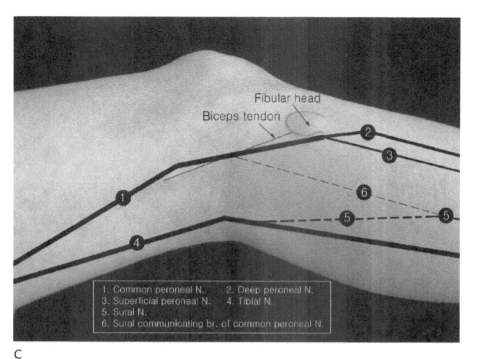

C

1. Common peroneal N.   2. Deep peroneal N.
3. Superficial peroneal N.   4. Tibial N.
5. Sural N.
6. Sural communicating br. of common peroneal N.

D

Figure 4-1. *(Continued)* **C:** *Anatomy of peroneal and tibial nerves at the knee.*
D: *Anatomy of the popliteal fossa and placement of stimulating electrodes.*

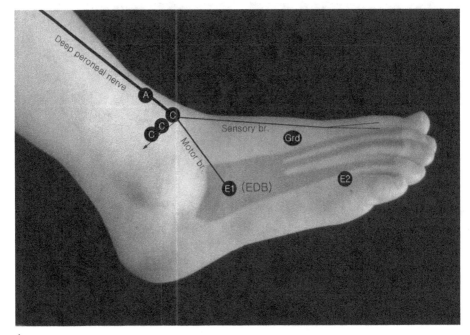

A

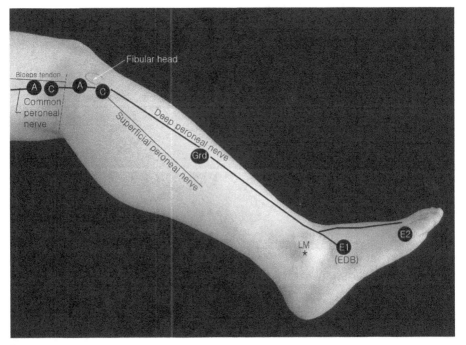

B

Figure 4-2. *A: Peroneal nerve motor conduction to the extensor digitorum brevis. B: Proximal stimulation sites in peroneal nerve motor conduction studies.*

Below fibular head: The nerve is stimulated just below and lateral to the fibular head.

Knee: The stimulation is applied at the cross-section point between the lateral hamstring tendon and crease of the popliteal fossa. Proximal to this point, it is often difficult to stimulate because the nerve is positioned more deeply under the biceps femoris tendon. Stimulation applied more proximal to the popliteal fossa may excite both the peroneal and tibial nerves because of both nerves' close proximity.

Reference Values

Distal latency [milliseconds (ms)]	Amplitude [millivolts (mV)]		Conduction velocity [meters per second (m/s)]
	A-BFH	AFH	
4.5 ± 0.8	4.4 ± 1.0	51.6 ± 4.1	53.9 ± 4.3

Comments While stimulating the nerve at the ankle, it is recommended that the cathode be applied just above the extensor retinaculum, considering the anterior tarsal tunnel syndrome, although it is rare.

ACCESSORY PERONEAL NERVE CONDUCTION STUDIES

(Fig. 4-3, Fig. 4-4)
Anomalous innervation to the extensor digitorum brevis occurs approximately 20% of the time. The accessory peroneal nerve, an extension of superficial peroneal nerve, courses posteriorly and under the lateral malleolus, where stimulation is applied. It is indicated by a different (smaller) compound muscle action potential (CMAP) (partial anomaly) or an absence of a CMAP (complete anomaly) when stimulating the deep peroneal nerve distally at the ankle.

PERONEAL MOTOR CONDUCTION STUDY TO THE TIBIALIS ANTERIOR

(Fig. 4-5A)

Tibialis Anterior Recording (Devi et al.)[2]

E1 The E1 electrode is placed at the junction of the upper one-third and lower two-thirds of a line between the tibial tuberosity and the tip of the lateral malleolus of the fibula.

E2 The E2 electrode is placed over the medial aspect of the tibia, 4 cm distal to the active electrode.

---

[2] Devi S, Lovelace RE, Duarte N: Proximal peroneal nerve conduction velocity: Recording from anterior tibial and peroneus brevis muscles. *Ann Neurol* 1979;2:116–119.

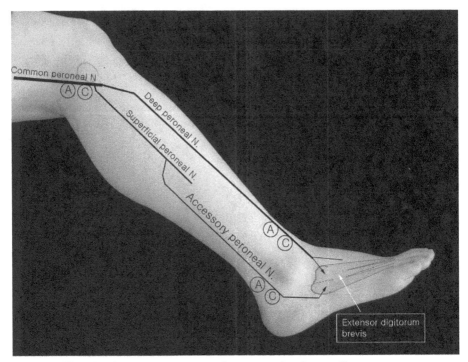

Figure 4-3. *Accessory peroneal nerve conduction studies.*

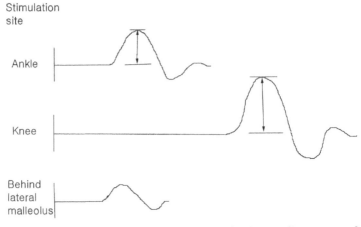

Figure 4-4. *Accessory peroneal nerve conduction studies. A part of the extensor digitorum brevis muscle is innervated by the accessory peroneal nerve.*

Stimulation

The stimulation is applied below the head of the fibula and the popliteal fossa along the medial border of the biceps femoris tendon with about 10 cm between the two points of stimulation.

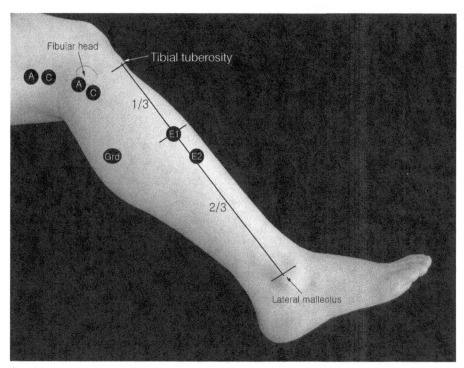

A

Figure 4-5. **A:** *Peroneal motor nerve conduction studies to the tibialis anterior (Devi et al).*[2]

PERONEAL MOTOR NERVE CONDUCTION TO THE TIBIALIS ANTERIOR AND PERONEUS LONGUS (LEE ET AL.)[3]

(Fig. 4-5B)

Tibialis Anterior

E1 The E1 electrode is placed on the belly of tibialis anterior, 8 cm distal to the fibular neck stimulation point.

E2 The E2 electrode is positioned over the tibialis anterior tendon at the ankle.

Peroneus Longus

E1 The E1 electrode is placed on a point on the proximal one-third of the peroneous longus/fibula, 8 cm distal to the fibular neck stimulation point.

E2 The E2 electrode is placed over the peroneus longus tendon at the ankle.

Stimulation Sites

Fibular neck, below fibular head.

Popliteal fossa

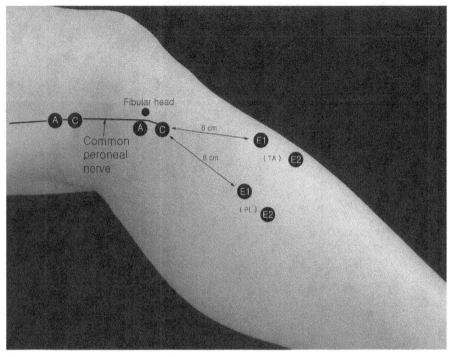

B

Figure 4-5. *(Continued)* **B:** *Peroneal motor nerve conduction studies to the tibialis anterior and peroneous longus (Lee et al.)*[3]

Reference Values

Devi et al.[2]

To tibialis anterior	Below fibular head	Above fibular head
Latency (ms)	3.0 ± 0.6	4.7 ± 0.5

Conduction velocity across the fibular head, 66.3 ± 12.9 (m per s)

Distance from point of stimulus to the E1 was not specified. Skin temperature also was not specified. However, the room was kept at a constant temperature of 22.2°C to 23.3°C.

Lee et al.[3] $N = 81$

Recording site	Latency (ms)	Amplitude (mV)
Tibialis anterior	2.5 ± 0.3	6.2 ± 1.3
	(3.6 to 9.3)	
Peroneus longus	2.6 ± 0.2	6.2 ± 1.4
	(3.4 to 10.6)	

---

[3] Lee HJ, Bach JR, DeLisa JA: Peroneal nerve motor conduction to the proximal muscles an alternative approach to conventional methods. *Am J Phys Med Rehabil* 1997;76:197–199.

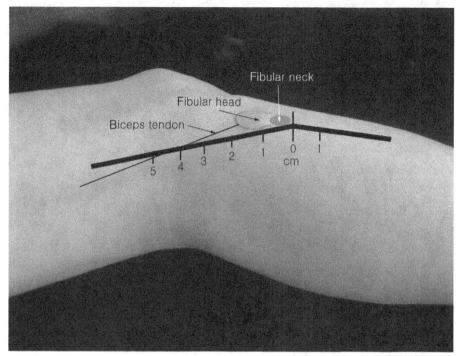

Figure 4-6. *Short segment incremental stimulation (SSIS) of the peroneal nerve across the fibular head.*

Comments Peroneal motor conduction to the tibialis anterior may be useful to assess the electrophysiogic abnormalities of the peroneal nerve when the motor response is absent because of severe atrophy of the extensor digitorum brevis. In common peroneal neuropathy at the knee, the superficial peroneal nerve often is less involved than the deep peroneal nerve. Thus, the CMAP recorded from the tibialis anterior may be a part of a volume-conducted response from the adjacent peroneus longus.

PERONEAL MOTOR NERVE CONDUCTION ACROSS THE KNEE: SHORT SEGMENT STIMULATION

(Fig. 4-6)

Recording Electrode Placement

E1 The E1 is placed over the belly of the extensor digitorum brevis.

E2 The E2 electrode is secured over the metatarsophalangeal joint of the little toe.

Stimulation

Stimulation is applied at 2-cm intervals along the path of the peroneal motor nerve across the fibular head.

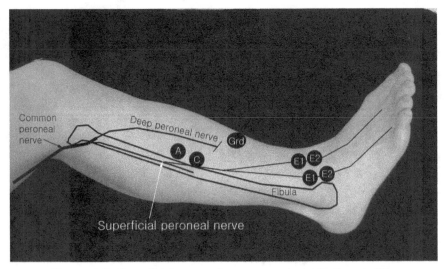

Figure 4-7. *Superficial peroneal nerve sensory conduction studies.*

Reference Values[4] $N = 46$

Conduction time at 2-cm intervals, 0.55 ± 0.1 ms

Amplitude changes, when compared with the succeeding distal responses at 2-cm intervals, $0.2 + 0.1$ mV.

SUPERFICIAL PERONEAL NERVE SENSORY CONDUCTION

(Fig. 4-7)

Recording Electrode Placements

The intermediate branch of the superficial peroneal nerve can be studied with E1 and E2 electrodes embedded in a plastic bar 1 to 2 cm medial to the lateral malleolus at the ankle. Slight repositioning of the bar electrode toward the tibialis anterior tendon may record the medial branch.

Stimulation

The stimulation is applied 12 to 14 cm proximal to the E1 electrode, just anterior to the anterior edge of the fibula. Occasionally, the stimulator may have to be firmly pressed against the skin. Slight repositioning of the original stimulation point proximally or distally may be required to elicit the optimal sensory response.

---

[4] Kanakamedala RV, Hong CZ: Peripheral nerve entrapment at the knee localized by short segment stimulation. *Am J Phys Med Rehabil* 1989;68:116–122.

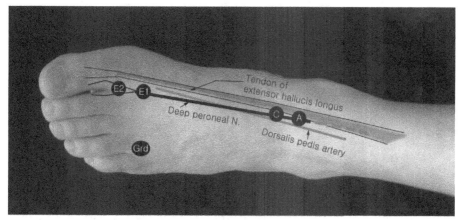

Figure 4-8. *Deep peroneal sensory nerve conduction studies.*

Reference Values

Jabre[5]—antidromic studies with 12 cm in distance.

Latency (ms)	Amplitude [microvolts (μV)]	Conduction velocity (m/s)
2.9 ± 0.3	20.5 ± 6.1	65.7 ± 3.7

Izzo et al.[6]—antidromic studies: distance, 14 cm. $N = 80$

	Latency (peak) (ms)	Amplitude (μV)	Conduction velocity (m/s)
Medial branch	3.4 ± 0.4	18.3 ± 8.0	51.2 ± 5.7
Intermediate branch	3.4 ± 0.4	15.1 ± 8.2	51.3 ± 5.4

DEEP PERONEAL SENSORY NERVE CONDUCTION STUDIES

(Fig. 4-8)

Recording Electrode Placements

E1 and E2 The E1 and E2 electrodes embedded in a plastic bar are placed at the first web space between the first and second metatarsal bones on the dorsum of the foot.

Stimulation

The stimulating cathode is placed near the dorsalis pedis (identified by palpation) near the ankle joint, just lateral to the extensor hallucis longus tendon and 8 to 10 cm proximal to the E1 recording electrode.

---

[5] Jabre JF: The superficial peroneal sensory nerve revisited. *Arch Neurol* 1981;38:666–667.
[6] Izzo KL, Sridhara CR, Lemont H, et al.: Sensory conduction studies of branches of the superficial peroneal nerve. *Arch Phys Med Rehabil* 1981;62:24–27.

Reference Values

Lee et al.[7]—antidromic studies: distance, 12 cm. $N = 40$

Latency (ms)		Amplitude (μV)	Conduction velocity (m/s)
Onset	Peak		
2.9 ± 0.4	3.6 ± 0.4	3.4 ± 1.4	42 ± 5

Posas et al.[8]—antidromic studies: distance, 10 cm. $N = 36$

Peak latency (ms)	Amplitude (μV)
3.2 ± 0.5	5.2 ± 0.5

Comments Because of the short distance between the stimulating and recording electrodes, shock artifacts are common in conduction studies. Applying small electric currents [e.g., 5 to 10 milliamperes (mA) with 0.1-ms pulse duration] and rotation of anode are often helpful. Occasionally, repositioning the cathode slightly lateral to the original stimulation point may enhance eliciting the sensory response because the nerve and dorsalis pedis artery may be displaced more laterally. A monopolar needle electrode (E1) with surface reference electrode (E2) can also be used. A side-to-side comparison is helpful.

PERONEAL MIXED NERVE CONDUCTION ACROSS THE FIBULAR HEAD

(Fig. 4-9)

Recording Electrode Placements

E1 and E2 electrodes embedded in a plastic bar are secured below and anterior to the fibular neck area.

Stimulation

The stimulation is applied at the intersection between the medial border of the biceps long head tendon and the popliteal crease.

Reference Values

Subject: 35 (70 nerves)

	Amplitude (μV)	Conduction velocity (m/s)
Right	24.8 ± 7.4	61.6 ± 4.5
Left	23.3 ± 6.9	61.7 ± 4.3

Values are means $\pm$ SD

---

[7] Lee HJ: Compound nerve action potential of common peroneal nerve recorded at fibular neck: its clinical usefulness. *Am J Phys Med Rehabil* 2001;80:108–112.

[8] Posas HN, Rivner MH: Nerve conduction studies of the medial branch of the deep peroneal nerve. *Muscle & Nerve* 1990;13:862.

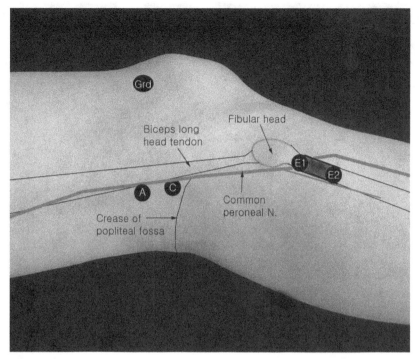

Figure 4-9. *Peroneal mixed nerve conduction studies across the fibular head.*

Comments Because of a short distance between the stimulating and recording electrodes, shock artifacts are troublesome. The recording electrodes are secured firmly with a wraparound Velcro strap.

LATERAL CUTANEOUS NERVE OF CALF CONDUCTION STUDIES (SURAL COMMUNICATING BRANCH OF COMMON PERONEAL NERVE)

(Fig. 4-10)

Recording Electrode Placements and Stimulation

Stimulation

A mark is made on the skin 2 cm behind the center of the fibular head and another is made 4 cm proximal to the first mark point.

E1 and E2 The E1 and E2 electrodes embedded in a plastic bar are placed 12 cm distal to the stimulation site in a line connecting the stimulation point and the tip of the calcaneus. Orthodromic conduction studies are also performed with the stimulating and recording electrodes were switched.

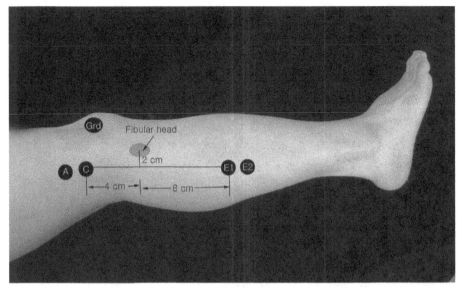

Figure 4-10. *Lateral cutaneous nerve of the calf (sural communicating branch of common peroneal nerve) conduction studies.*

Reference Values[9]

	Latency (ms)		Amplitude (μV)	Conduction velocity (m/s)
	Onset	Peak		
Antidromic	2.1 ± 0.3	2.6 ± 0.4	4.3 ± 2.5	60 ± 10
Orthodromic	2.3 ± 0.3	2.7 ± 0.3	5.0 ± 2.2	52 ± 5

Comments Of 64 limbs, the sensory response was recordable in 62 limbs with either antidromic or orthodromic studies.

 Tibial Nerve

TIBIAL MOTOR NERVE MOTOR CONDUCTION STUDIES

There are two recording sites in the foot muscles for recording a CMAP with stimulation of medial and lateral plantar branches (nerve) of the tibial nerve. Routine tibial motor conduction studies are performed with the medial plantar branch.

---

[9] Campagnolo DI, Romello MA, Park YI, Foye PM, DeLisa JA: Technique for studying in the lateral cutaneous nerve of calf. *Muscle & Nerve* 2000;23:1277–1279.

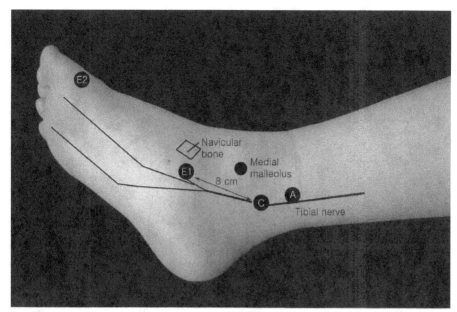

A

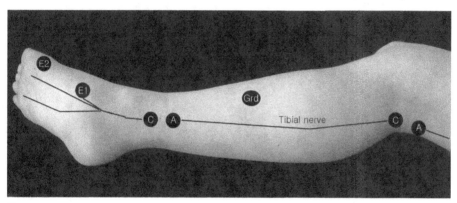

B

Figure 4-11. *A: Tibial nerve motor conduction studies to the abductor hallucis. B: Stimulation sites on tibial nerve motor conduction studies.*

MEDIAL PLANTAR NERVE CONDUCTION TO THE ABDUCTOR HALLUCIS

(Fig. 4-11, Fig. 4-12)

Recording Electrode Placement

E1 is placed 1 cm below and 1 cm behind the navicular tubercle on the medial side of the foot.

E2 is placed distally over the metatarsal-phalangeal joint of the great toe.

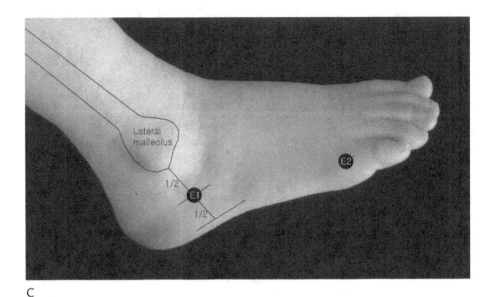

C

Figure 4-11. *(Continued) **C:** Tibial nerve conduction studies to the abductor digiti minimi.*

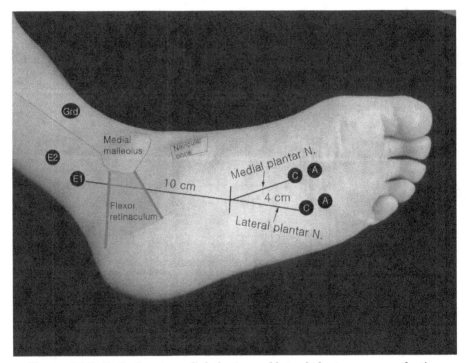

Figure 4-12. *Orthodromic medial plantar and lateral plantar nerve conduction studies.*

Stimulation Sites

Ankle: A stimulating cathode is placed posterior and just proximal to the medial malleolus, halfway between the medial malleolus and Achilles tendon.

Knee: Stimulate slightly lateral to the halfway point of the popliteal fossa along the popliteal crease.

Recommended Position for Stimulation

Ankle, neutral position

Knee, prone or side lying position

LATERAL PLANTAR NERVE TO THE ABDUCTOR DIGITI MINIMI

Recording Electrode Placement

E1 is placed directly below the lateral malleolus, bisecting the distance from the tip of the lateral malleolus to the sole of the foot.

E2 is secured over the metatarsal-phalangeal joint of the little toe.

Stimulation Sites

The same sites, ankle and knee, as that of medial plantar nerve are used for lateral plantar nerve.

Reference Values[10] ($N = 37$ adults)·

	Distal latency (ms)		Amplitude	Conduction velocity
Nerve	8 cm	10 cm	(mV)	(m/s)
Medial plantar	3.4 ± 0.5	3.8 ± 0.5	11.6 ± 4.3	54.9 ± 7.6
Lateral plantar	3.6 ± 0.5	3.9 ± 0.5		51.2 ± 3.9

Comments Distal distance (E1 to cathode) is measured the medial plantar nerve following the course of the nerve. A distance of 8 or 10 cm can be used, with stimulation applied posterior to the medial malleolus and above the flexor retinaculum. To ensure supramaximal stimulation at the popliteal fossa, higher stimulation intensities are needed. CMAP often is significantly lower with popliteal stimulation than with ankle stimulation. Thus, care must be taken whenever calling a conduction block of the tibial motor nerve between the popliteal fossa and ankle. Side-to-side comparison of the CMAPs might be useful. If a cathode is placed too laterally and higher stimulation currents are applied, a coactivation of both the tibial and peroneal nerves are possible. The CMAPs to

---

[10] Fu R, DeLisa JA, Kraft GH: Motor conduction latencies through the tarsal tunnel in normal adult subjects: Standard determinations corrected for temperature and distance. *Arch Phys Med Rehabil* 1980;61:243–248.

[11] Jimenez J, Easton JK, Redford JB: Conduction studies of the anterior and posterior tibial nerves. *Arch Phys Med Rehabil* 1970;51:164–169.

ankle and popliteal fossa stimulation must be the same shape. Skin temperature was measured below the medial malleolus, and the temperature range was 29°C to 34°C (mean, 32.1°C ± 1.4°C). The article of Fu et al.[10] has a table of temperature correction, as well as values obtained using calipers instead of flexible caliper.

MEDIAL AND LATERAL PLANTAR NERVES—COMPOUND (MIXED) NERVE ACTION POTENTIAL

(Fig. 4-12)

Recording Electrode Placements

E1 and E2 embedded in a bar electrode are placed behind the medial malleolus and proximal to the upper border of the flexor retinaculum.

Stimulation

The stimulating point for the medial plantar nerve is determined by first measuring 10 cm distal to the E1 electrode in the interspace between the first and second metatarsal bones on the sole and extended 4 cm distally. The lateral plantar nerve is stimulated 4 cm directly lateral to the 10-cm site of the medial plantar nerve. The medial and lateral plantar nerves are stimulated on the sole at a site 14 cm distal to E1, active recording electrode, over the corresponding nerves.

Electromyography (EMG) Machine Settings

Filters: 8 Hz to 1.6 kHz

Sweep speed: 5 msec/div

Sensitivity: 2 uV/div

Pulse duration: 0.2 msec

Reference Values[13]

Nerve	Latency to the negative peak (ms) (mean ± SD)	Amplitude (μV)
Medial plantar	3.2 ± 0.3 (range, 2.6 to 3.7)	>10 μV (range, 10 to 30)
Lateral plantar	3.2 ± 0.3 (range, 2.7 to 3.7)	>8 μV (range, 8 to 20)

Comments High stimulation currents with a long pulse duration are often required to evoke the mixed nerve potentials, especially in individuals with thick sole skin. Also, slight movements of the cathode medially or laterally and proximally or distally are needed to stimulate the nerves. The mean temperatures

---

[13] Saeed MA, Gatens PF: Compound nerve action potentials in the medial and lateral plantar nerves through tarsal tunnel. *Arch Phys Med Rehabil* 1982;63:304–307.

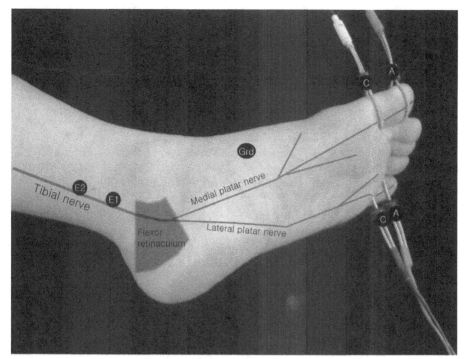

Figure 4-13. *Medial and lateral plantar nerve conduction studies.*

were as follows: tarsal tunnel, 30.7°C; medial sole, 29.8°C; lateral sole, 29.2°C. The distance is measured with a flexible metal tape.

MEDIAL AND LATERAL PLANTAR NERVES—ORTHODROMIC NERVE CONDUCTION STUDIES

(Fig. 4-13)

Recording Electrode Placement

A bar electrode is placed behind and just above the medial malleolus (flexor retinaculum).

Stimulating Electrodes

Medial plantar nerve, ring electrodes are applied on the great toe with anode distal.

Lateral plantar nerve, ring electrodes are placed on the fifth digit with anode distal.

Distance

No specific standard distance was noted.

Reference Values[14] ($N = 20$)

	Conduction velocity (m/s) (mean $\pm$ SD)	Amplitude (μV) (mean amplitude)
Medial plantar nerve	35.2 $\pm$ 3.6	3.6 (range, 2 to 6)
Lateral plantar nerve	31.7 $\pm$ 4.4	1.9 (range, 1 to 5)

(Latency is measured to the negative peak.)

Comments In young individuals, the sensory response can be obtained without averaging. Because of the small sensory response, signal averaging is required in most cases. The test is useful for confirmation of tarsal tunnel syndrome.

 Sural Nerve

(Fig. 4-14, Fig. 4-15)

Recording Electrode Placements for Antidromic Method

E1 The surface E1 electrode is placed posterior to and at the level of the neck of the lateral malleolus of the fibula.

E2 The E2 electrode is placed 3 to 4 cm distal to the E1.

Stimulation

The stimulating cathode with anode proximal is applied slightly lateral to the midline in the lower one-third of the posterior aspect of the leg. Site 10, 14, or 17 cm from the E1 is stimulated.

EMG Machine Settings

Filters, 20 Hz to 2 kHz

Sweep speed, 1 to 2 ms/div

Sensitivity, 10 μV

Duration of pulse, 0.1 to 0.2 ms

Measurement Parameters

Latency: To the negative peak or onset

Amplitude: Baseline-to-negative peak or peak-to-peak

Duration

---

[14] Oh SJ, Sarala PK, Kuba T, Elmore RS: Tarsal tunnel syndrome: Electrophysiological study. *Arch Neurol* 1979;5:327–330.

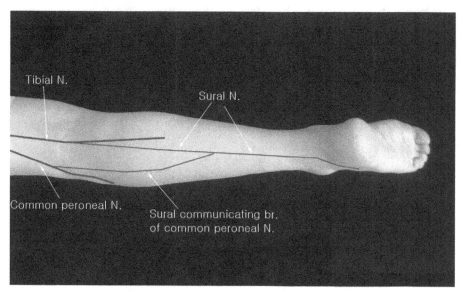

Figure 4-14. *Anatomy of the sural nerve.*

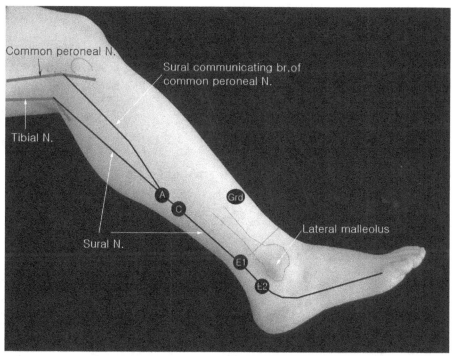

Figure 4-15. *Sural nerve conduction studies.*

Comments Patient lying on the side, with the testing extremity on top, is best for both the patient and examiner. The cathode may be shifted either laterally or medially to evoke an optimum sensory response. Also, the recording electrodes may have to be repositioned to optimize the sensory response, if the expected response is lower than normal. Because the nerve is superficial, it is activated easily without applying firm pressure to the skin. An audio system of the EMG machine may help to approximate the closeness of stimulation to the testing nerve. The patient feels shocks radiate to the lateral side of the heel and foot.

Reference Values

Schuchmann[15]

Latency to the negative peak

Distance (cm)	Latency (ms) (mean ± SD)	Number (N) of patients
10	3.8 ± 0.3	37
14	3.5 ± 0.3	56
17	4.0 ± 0.3	56
20	4.6 ± 0.4	54

Sensory potential, 5~ 30 uV

Korea University Medical Center **(KUMC)** (unpublished)

Age group (year)	Latency (ms) (mean ± SD)		Amplitude (µV) (mean ± SD)	N
	Peak	Onset		
21 to 30	3.4 ± 0.4	2.7 ± 0.2	22.3 ± 7.2	44
31 to 40	3.4 ± 0.2	2.7 ± 0.2	21.4 ± 6.9	34
41 to 50	3.3 ± 0.3	2.7 ± 0.3	19.4 ± 6.9	77
51 to 60	3.4 ± 0.3	2.7 ± 0.2	15.6 ± 5.8	64
61 to 70	3.4 ± 0.4	2.7 ± 0.4	13.6 ± 5.0	58
71 +	3.4 ± 0.3	2.7 ± 0.3	11.5 ± 4.4	24
All ages	**3.4 ± 0.3**	**2.7 ± 0.3**	**17.5 ± 7.2**	**301**

Comments: Antidromic study, 14 cm between the E1 electrode and the cathode. Skin temperature at ankle 30°C or higher.

Femoral Nerve Motor Conduction Studies

(Fig. 4-16, Fig. 4-17)

VASTUS MEDIALIS RECORDINGS

E1 The E1 electrode, either surface or needle, is placed over the belly of the vastus medialis.

---

15 Schuchmann JA: Sural nerve conduction: A standardized technique. *Arch Phys Med Rehabil* 1977; 58:166–168.

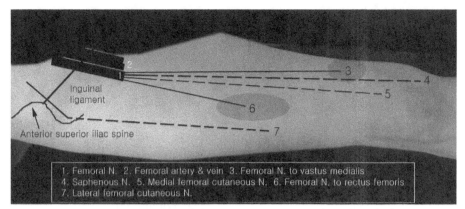

1. Femoral N. 2. Femoral artery & vein 3. Femoral N. to vastus medialis
4. Saphenous N. 5. Medial femoral cutaneous N. 6. Femoral N. to rectus femoris
7. Lateral femoral cutaneous N.

Figure 4-16. *Anatomy of inguinal area—anterior thigh and nerve.*

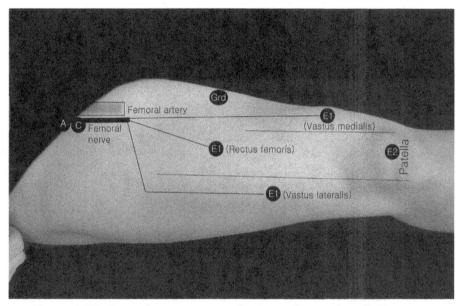

Figure 4-17. *Femoral nerve motor conduction to the vastus medialis, vastus lateralis, and rectus femoris.*

E2 The reference electrode is attached to the tendon of the vastus medialis tendon near the medial proximal border of the patella.

RECTUS FEMORIS RECORDINGS

E1 The E1 electrode is positioned over the belly of rectus femoris, 14 and 30 cm from stimulation.

E2 The E2 electrode is placed over the tendon of the rectus femoris near the patella.

Stimulation

The stimulating cathode is placed just below the inguinal ligament and lateral to the femoral artery.

Reference Values

Gassel[16]

A concentric needle electrode was inserted in the vastus medialis and lateralis and rectus femoris. No difference was noted in the latency or conduction velocity measurement between placement in three different muscles if distance was kept constant. $N = 40$

Latency (ms)		Mean conduction velocity (m/s)
14 cm	30 cm	
3.7 ± 0.1	6.0 ± 0.2	70 ± 7.8*

*Mean conduction velocity calculated between 14- and 30-cm points.

Johnson et al.[17]

Surface pickups were used, with the E1 electrode placed over the vastus medialis. Needle electrode tends to facilitate stimulation of the femoral nerve.

Stimulation site	Latency (ms)
Above the inguinal ligament	7.1 ± 0.7 (6.1 to 8.4)
Below the inguinal ligament	6.0 ± 0.7 (5.5 to 7.5)
Delay across the inguinal ligament	1.1 ± 0.4 (0.8 to 1.8)

Comments Side-to-side comparisons of the latencies and compound muscle action potential amplitudes are useful to assess electrophysiologic abnormalities in femoral neuropathy.

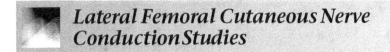

Lateral Femoral Cutaneous Nerve Conduction Studies

(Fig. 4-18)

Recording Electrode Placements

E1 A line can be made with a tape measure between the anterior superior iliac spine and the lateral border of the patella. On that line, the E1 electrode is placed 16 and 18 cm from the anterior superior iliac spine.

E2 The E2 electrode is placed 4 cm distal to the E1.

[16] Gassel MM: A study of femoral nerve conduction time. *Arch Neurol* 1963;9:607–614.
[17] Johnson EW, Wood PK, Power JJ: Femoral nerve conduction studies. *Arch Phys Med Rehabil* 1968;49:528–532.

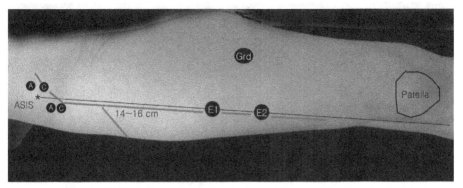

Figure 4-18. *Lateral femoral cutaneous nerve conduction studies.*

Stimulation

The stimulating electrodes, either surface or monopolar needle, are placed 1 cm medial to the anterior superior iliac spine. Because of a small sensory potential, the points of stimulation are repositioned more distally near the proximal lateral border of the sartorius. The recording electrodes have to be repositioned either laterally or medially. Reducing the electrical shock artifacts may require a rotation of the anode to the cathode or use of small currents with a short pulse duration.

Reference Values

Butler[18] $N = 24$ Distance $= 12$ cm

Latency (negative peak) (ms)	Amplitude (μV)	Conduction velocity (m/s)
2.6 ± 0.2	10 to 25	47.9 ± 3.7

Comments Recording the lateral femoral cutaneous nerve is technically very difficult especially in individuals with obesity.

Posterior Femoral Cutaneous Nerve Conduction Studies

(Fig. 4-19)

Recording Electrode Placements

E1 The E1 electrode is placed in the midline of the posterior thigh 6 cm proximal to the crease of the popliteal fossa.

E2 The reference electrode is located 4 cm distal the E1 electrode.

---

[18] Butler ET, Johnson EW: Normal conduction velocity in the lateral femoral cutaneous nerve. *Arch Phys Med Rehabil* 1974;55:31–32.

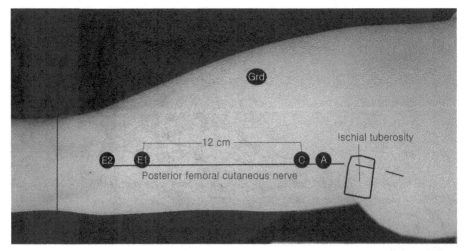

Figure 4-19. *Posterior femoral cutaneous nerve conduction studies.*

Stimulation

The stimulating cathode is placed 12 cm proximal, in a line connecting the E1 recording electrode and the ischial tuberosity and in the groove between the medial and lateral hamstrings.

Reference Values

Dumitru[19] $N = 80$, Age 20 to 78 (mean 34)

Latency to negative peak (ms)	Amplitude (μV)
2.8 ± 0.2	6.5 ± 1.5

 ## Medial Femoral Cutaneous Nerve Conduction Studies

Recording Electrode Placements

E1 With a tape measure, a line connecting the femoral artery identified by a pulsation at the inguinal area and medial border of the patella can be made. The E1 electrode is placed above the noted line 14 to 16 cm distal from the inguinal area, just lateral to the femoral artery.

E2 The E2 electrode is placed 4 cm distal to the E1 active recording electrode.

---

[19] Dumitru D, Nelson MR: Posterior femoral cutaneous nerve conduction. *Arch Phys Med Rehabil* 1990;71:979–982.

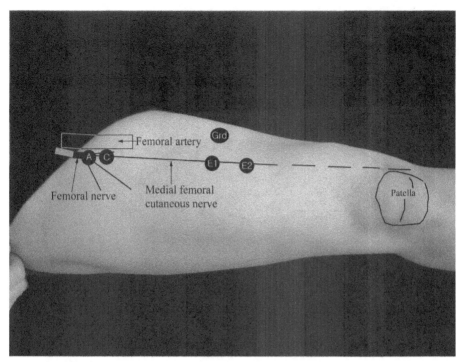

Figure 4-20. *Medial femoral cutaneous nerve conduction studies.*

Stimulation

The stimulation with firm pressure is applied just lateral to the femoral artery pulsation 2 to 4 cm below the inguinal ligament. At this point, direct stimulation of the femoral nerve can be eliminated.

Reference Values

Lee et al.[20]

Subjects = 35 (70 nerves)	Mean ± SD
Onset latency (ms)	2.4 ± 0.2
Peak latency (ms)	2.9 ± 0.3
Nerve conduction velocity (NCV) (m/s)	60 ± 5.0
Amplitude (μV)	4.8 ± 1.0

Comments Because of small potentials, repositioning the cathode and recording electrodes placed slightly medially or laterally from the original sites is required.

---

[20] Lee HJ, Bach JR, DeLisa JA: Medial femoral cutaneous nerve conduction. *Am J Phys Med Rehabil* 1995;74:305–307.

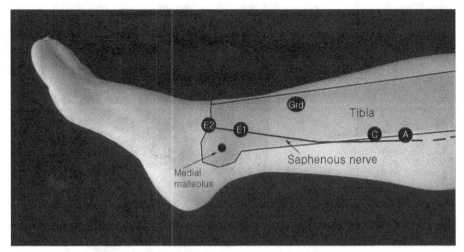

Figure 4-21. *Saphenous nerve conduction studies.*

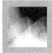

Saphenous Nerve Conduction Studies

(Fig. 4-21)

Recording Electrode Placements

E1 and E2 The E1 active recording and E2 reference electrodes embedded in a bar are placed at the ankle with the E2 electrode positioned anteriorly to the prominence of the medial malleolus. The E1 electrode is located proximally to the E2 electrode between the anterior border of the tibia and tibialis anterior tendon.

Stimulation

Antidromic stimulation is performed 12 to 14 cm from the E1 recording electrode, deep to the medial border of the tibia. Firm pressure is applied, pushing the stimulator between the medial border of the tibia and medial gastrocnemius muscle.

Reference Values[21] $N = 40$

Latency (negative peak) (ms)	Amplitude (μV)	Conduction velocity (m/s)
3.6 ± 0.4	9.0 ± 3.4	41.7 ± 3.4

---

[21] Wainapel SF, Kim DJ, Ebel A: Conduction studies of the saphenous nerve in healthy subjects. *Arch Phys Med Rehabil* 1978;59:316–319.

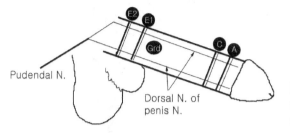

Pudendal N.

Dorsal N. of
penis N.

Figure 4-22. *Dorsal nerve of the penis nerve conduction studies.*

Dorsal Nerve of the Penis

(Fig. 4-22)

Recording Electrode Placements

E1 The **E1** ring electrode is placed at the most proximal base of the penis.

E2 The **E2** ring electrode is placed proximal to the E1 electrode on the penis or a surface E2 electrode is placed 4 cm proximal to the E1 above the symphysis pubis.

Stimulation

The stimulating cathode electrode is placed just proximal to the dorsal glans with the anode distal on the dorsal glans.

EMG Machine Settings

Same as routine sensory conduction studies.

Reference Values[22] $N = 20$

NCV, 36.2 ± 3.2 m/s

Latency, 2.3 ± 0.4 ms

Amplitude, 2.3 ± 1.1 μV

Comments This is an orthodromic conduction study and the mean skin temperature measured from the midshaft of the penis was 31.8°C (range, 30°C to 33.5°C). The interelectrode distance ranged from 5.4 to 11.5 cm (mean ± SD, 8.6 ± 1.5 cm). Sensory Nerve Action Potential (SNAP) amplitude is small. A penile traction device was used. Conduction velocities are different depending whether the penis shaft is flaccid or stretched. The test may be useful to assess the penile sensory component in erectile dysfunction.

---

[22] Clawson DR, Cardenas DD: Dorsal nerve of the penis conduction velocity: A new technique. *Muscle & Nerve* 1991;14:845–849.

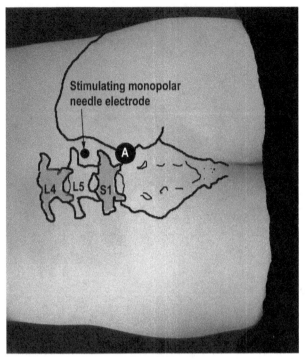

Figure 4-23. *L5 and S1 spinal root stimulation and conduction studies.*

L5 and S1 Spinal Root Stimulations

(Fig. 4-23, Fig. 4-24)

Recording Electrode Placements

Recording (active E1 and reference E2) electrodes are placed over the tibialis anterior, abductor hallucis, soleus and flexor pollicis brevis, etc.

Stimulation

A monopolar needle (Teflon coated) is inserted about 1 cm medial and slightly caudal to the posterior superior iliac spine. The same type of needle is placed on the opposite side in an identical manner. A 50- to 75-mm needle is required. The anode (surface electrode) is placed on the anterior abdomen just opposite the needle electrode or it is placed over the spinous process.

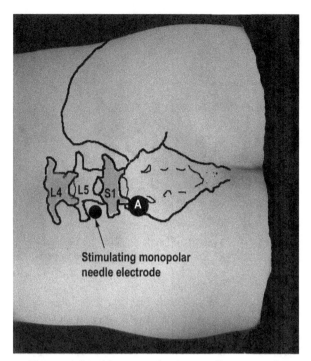

Figure 4-24. *Motor conduction studies across the sacral plexus.*

Reference Values

Kraft[23]

Conduction latency to the soleus, 15.4 ± 1.3 ms

Side-to-side difference, 0.2 ms (range, 0 to 0.8 ms)

MacDonell[24]

Needle electrode stimulation was compared with magnetic coil stimulation in the lumbosacral nerve root. With both techniques, the latency did not differ significantly.

Conduction latency to the tibialis anterior, 13.5 ± 1.2 ms (range, 11.4 to 15.9)

Conduction latency to the flexor pollicis brevis, 25.1 ± 2.0 ms (range, 21.7 to 29.7)

[23] Kraft GH, Johnson EW: *Proximal nerve conduction and late responses.* American Association of Electromyography and Electrodiagnosis Workshop, Sept. 1986.
[24] MacDonell RA, Cros D, Shahani BT: Lumbosacral nerve root stimulation comparing electrical with surface magnetic coil techniques. *Muscle & Nerve* 1992;15:885–890.

Motor Conduction Studies Across the Sacral Plexus

(Fig. 4-24)

Recording Electrode Placements

E1 The E1 electrode is placed over the belly of the abductor hallucis.

E2 The E2 electrode is placed near the first metatarsal bone.

Stimulation

Proximal: The L5 or S1 root is stimulated by a monopolar needle electrode (cathode) inserted about 1 cm medial and slightly caudal to the posterior superior iliac spine. The anode is a surface electrode placed over the spinous process.

Distal To measure conduction across the sacral plexus, the sciatic nerve is stimulated with the same monopolar needle electrode, inserting it at the gluteal skin fold midway between the greater trochanter of the femur and the ischial tuberosity. The anode is a surface electrode attached near the needle electrode.

Reference Values

Latency across the sacral plexus, 3.9 ± 0.7 ms (range, 2.5 to 4.9)

Side-to-side difference, 0 to 1.0 ms

Sciatic Motor Nerve Conduction Study

(Fig. 4-25)

Recording Electrode Placements

E1 The E1 electrode is placed over abductor digiti minimi.

E2 The E2 reference electrode is attached on the little toe.

Stimulation

Proximal stimulation: A Teflon-coated monopolar needle electrode is inserted midway between the ischial tuberosity and the greater trochanter of the femur.

Distal stimulation: Surface electrode stimulators are applied at the popliteal fossa.

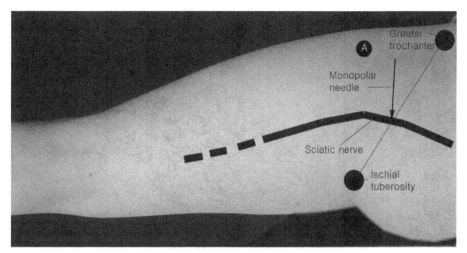

Figure 4-25. *Sciatic motor nerve conduction studies.*

Reference Values

Yap[25] $N = 10$

Velocity, 51.3 ± 4.4 m/s (range, 45.3 to 61.1) to abductor digiti minimi.

Comments The sciatic nerve is vulnerable to entrapment as it crosses the sciatic notch in leaving the pelvis.

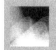

Bulbocavernosus Reflex—Pudendal Nerve

(Fig. 4-26)

Recording Electrode Placements

The recording electrode is a *standard concentric needle* inserted into the bulbocavernosus muscle. This muscle is superficial and is located under the scrotum on both sides of the midline. Needle placement can be confirmed by squeezing the glans penis and observing the bulbocavernosus reflex. A monopolar needle also can be inserted into the bulbocavernosus muscle. A surface electrode as referenced is placed near the monopolar needle.

---

[25] Yap CB, Hirota T: Sciatic nerve motor conduction velocity study. *J Neurol Neurosurg Psychiatry* 1967;30:233–239.

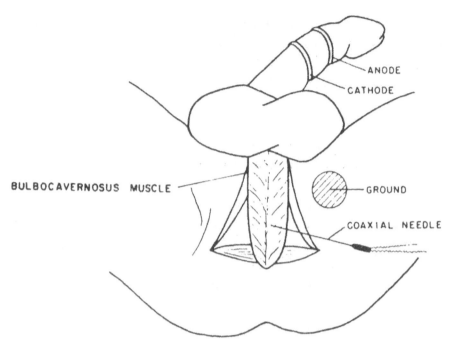

Figure 4-26. *Bulbocavernosus reflex studies.*

Stimulation

Ring electrodes of a stimulator are placed on the penile shaft with the cathode proximal.

EMG Machine Settings

Filters, 8 Hz to 8 kHz

Sweep speed, 10 ms/div

Sensitivity, 200 μV/div

Pulse duration, 0.1 ms

Reference Values

Siroky[26] N = 52

Latency to the negative peak, 35 $\pm$ 2 ms (range, 28 to 42)

Dick[27] N = 10

Average latency, 31 ms (range, 24 to 40)

---

[26] Siroky MB, Sax DS, Krane RJ: Sacral signal tracing: The electrophysiology of the bulbocavernosus reflex. *J Urol* 1979;122:661–664.

[27] Dick HC, Bradley WE, Scott FB, Timm GW: Pudendal sxual reflex. Electrophysiologic investigation. *Urology* 1979;3:376–379.

Comments This study also can be done on women. Either the clitoris is stimulated or a special stimulator is attached to a Foley catheter and placed intraurethrally. It appears that 42 ms is normal with various techniques.

 Abbreviations

ms, milliseconds; mV, millivolts; m per s, meters per second; CMAP, compound muscle action potential; μV, microvolts; mA, milliamperes; EMG, electromyography; cm, centimeters; NCV, nerve conduction velocity.

CHAPTER 5

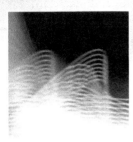

Proximal Nerve Conduction Studies in Upper Extremity and Cervical Plexus

Surface Anatomy and Brachial Plexus Stimulation at Erb's Point

(Fig. 5-1, Fig. 5-2)

The brachial plexus lies in the supraclavicular fossa, between the clavicle and the lower part of the posterior border of the sternocleidomastoid. It emerges between the scalenus anterior and scalenus medius. When the arm is by the side, the plexus can be felt as a bunch of tense cords with a relative firm press by a finger tip 2 to 3 centimeters (cm) proximal to the anterior convexity of the medial two-thirds of the clavicle. This area may match with Erb's point, a point 2 or 3 cm above the clavicle and beyond the posterior border of the sternocleidomastoid, at the level of the transverse process of the sixth cervical vertebra. The stimulating cathode placed at this point can stimulate the brachial plexus. The patient's head can be turned to the opposite side of stimulation. The stimulation site is identified when the patient notes discomfort with firm pressure over the plexus. Because the brachial plexus is crossed by many different structures (arterys, veins, muscles, and nerves other than plexus) at this point, supramaximal stimulation is often difficult to achieve, requiring high current intensities with a long duration of pulse. Stimulation at Erb's point can stimulate the entire brachial plexus, not an individual nerve, so some degree of a volume-conducted muscle response from adjacent muscles may be inevitable.

Distance Measurement

Accurate measurement of distance between the stimulation and recording points in proximal motor conduction is often difficult and inaccurate. Measurements

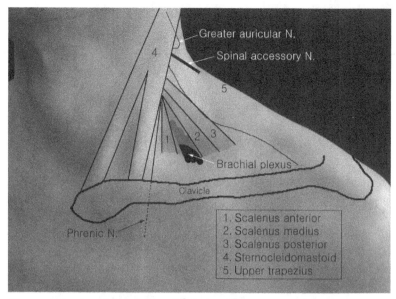

Figure 5-1. *Anatomy of supraclavicular fossa and brachial plexus.*

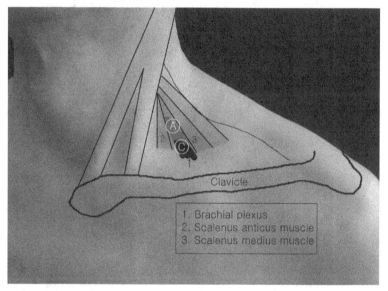

Figure 5-2. *Brachial plexus stimulation point at the supraclavicular fossa/Erb's point stimulation.*

with an obstetrical caliper is best, although a flexible tape can be used. Most previous tests were done with unfixed distances.

Recommendation for the Conduction Studies

Side-to-side comparisons of latency and amplitude are very useful in diagnosing lesions of proximal nerves.

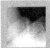

Axillary Nerve Conduction to the Deltoid

(Fig. 5-3)

Recording Electrode Placements

E1 A surface electrode is placed over the most prominent portion of the middle deltoid muscle. A monopolar needle can also be used as the E1 electrode.

E2 Using a surface electrode, the E2 electrode is attached over the insertion of the deltoid, approximately midway in the humerus.

Stimulation

The cathode is placed in the supraclavicular fossa, just lateral to the sternocleido-mastoid muscle. The anode is positioned proximal to the cathode. Stimulation

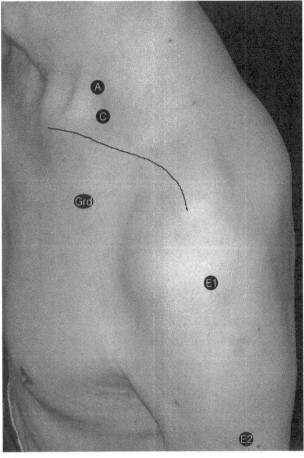

Figure 5-3. *Axillary nerve conduction studies to the deltoid muscle.*

applied at Erb's point stimulates the brachial plexus (trunk—upper, middle, and lower). Firm pressure applied at Erb's point and a long-pulse duration [~1 millisecond (ms)] by the stimulator are often necessary to evoke an optimal compound muscle action potential (CMAP).

Reference Values $N = 62$

Latency, 3.9 ± 0.5 ms (range, 2.8 to 5.0)

Distance, range, 14.8 to 26.5 cm

Comments For distance measurement, a flexible tape can be used, but obstetrical calipers are more accurate than the tape. Side-to-side comparisons of latency and amplitude are useful. [1]

Musculocutaneous Nerve Conduction to the Biceps Brachii

(Fig. 5-4)

Recording Electrode Placements

E1 The E1 active recording electrode is placed over the most prominent muscle belly (midpoint) of the biceps brachii.

E2 The E2 reference electrode is positioned at the tendon of the biceps brachii at the elbow.

Stimulation

Supraclavicular fossa (see page 100 for details)

Reference Values[1] $N = 62$

Latency, 4.5 ± 0.6 ms (range, 3.3 to 5.7)

Distance, range, 23.5 to 41.5 cm[1]

Suprascapular Nerve to the Supraspinatus and Infraspinatus Muscles

SUPRASPINATUS MUSCLE RECORDING

1. A standard concentric needle is inserted medial to the midpoint of the scapular spine and just above the spine. It is directed in a downward and

---

[1] Kraft GH: Axillary, musculocuataneous and suprascapular nerve latency studies. *Arch Phys Med Rehabil* 1972;53:383–387.

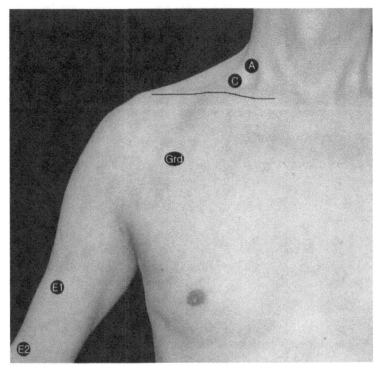

Figure 5-4. *Musculocutaneous nerve conduction studies to the biceps brachii.*

anterior direction until bone contact is made, and then the needle is withdrawn slightly. Shoulder abduction may confirm the needle placement. The study is done with patients either sitting or side-lying with arms at the side.

2.   A monopolar needle can be used with a surface electrode as the E2 reference electrode. The needle is inserted as described above.

INFRASPINATUS MUSCLE RECORDING
(Fig. 5-5)
Surface or needle electrodes can be used. The surface E1 electrode is placed several centimeters lateral to the medial border of the scapula and 2 to 3 cm below the scapular spine. The E2 surface electrode is positioned 2 cm more distal to the stimulating cathode. Also, needle electrodes may be used as above noted.

Reference Values $N = 62$

Latency to	Latency (ms)	Distance
Supraspinatus	2.7 ± 0.5 (1.7 to 3.7)	range, 7.4 to 13.8 cm
Infraspinatus	3.3 ± 0.5 (2.4 to 4.2)	range, 10.6 to 19.5 cm[1]

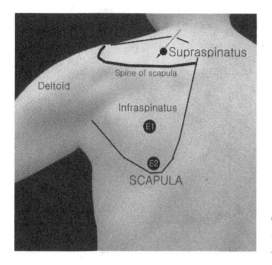

Figure 5-5. *Suprascapular nerve conduction studies to the supraspinatus and infraspinatus muscles with Erb's point stimulation.*

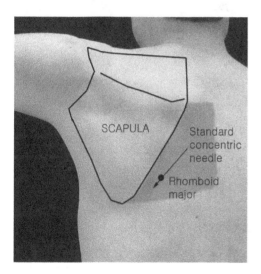

Figure 5-6. *Dorsal scapular nerve conduction studies to the rhomboid.*

 Dorsal Scapular Nerve to the Rhomboid Muscle

(Fig. 5-6)

Recording Electrode Placements

A standard concentric needle is inserted into the rhomboid major muscle at the medial edge of the inferior angle of the scapula.

Stimulation

Surface electrode stimulator is placed at Erb's point.

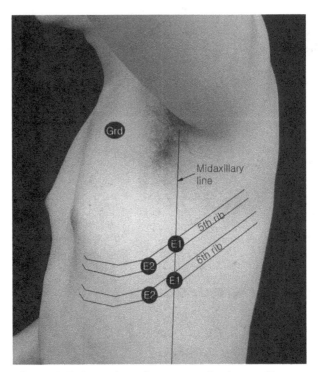

Figure 5-7. *Long thoracic nerve conduction studies to the serratus anterior.*

Reference Values[2] $N = 21$ Age, mean $= 42.3$ years (19 to 73)

Latency, 5.2 ± 0.7 ms

Distance, 16.5 to 21.5 cm[2]

 ## Long Thoracic Nerve to the Serratus Anterior

(Fig. 5-7)

Recording Electrode Placements

E1 and E2 Surface recording electrodes are used. The E1 electrode is placed over the fifth or sixth rib at the midaxillary line. The E2 electrode is positioned on the same rib 3 to 4 cm more anteriorly then the E1 electrode. When needle electrode recording is performed, care must be taken not to inadvertently pierce the intercostal space, producing pneumothorax.

Stimulation

The stimulation is given at Erb's point.

[2] Lo Monaco M, Di Pasqua PG, Tonali P: Conduction studies along the accessory, long thoracic, dorsal scapular, and thoracodorsal nerves. *Acta Neurol Scand* 1983;68:171–176.

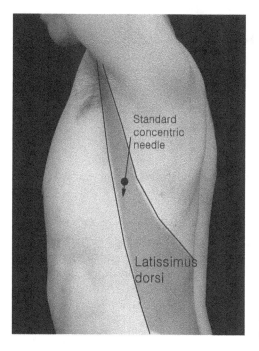

Figure 5-8. *Thoracodorsal nerve conduction studies to the latissimus dorsi.*

Reference Values $N = 25$

Latency, 3.9 ± 0.6 ms

(monopolar needle electrode recordings)[3]

Thoracodorsal Nerve to the Latissimus Dorsi

(Fig. 5-8)

Recording Electrode Placements

A standard concentric needle electrode is inserted into the belly of the latissimus dorsi at the posterior wall of the axilla.

Stimulation

Stimulation is performed at Erb's point with a surface stimulator.

Reference Values[3] $N = 19$ Age, 22 to 73

Latency, 3.9 ± 0.4 ms

Distance, 17 to 21 cm^2

---

[3] Kaplan PE: Electrodiagnostic confirmation of long thoracic nerve palsy. *J Neurol Neurosurg Psychiatry* 1980;43:50–52.

Phrenic Nerve Conduction Studies to the Diaphragm

(Fig. 5-9)

Recording Electrode Placements

The active recording electrode E1 is placed at the xyphoid process. The E2 reference electrodes are attached at the seventh intercostal space bilaterally.

Stimulation

The surface stimulating electrode is placed at the posterior border of the sternocleidomastoid muscle at the level of the thyroid cartilage. Alternatively, the cathode can also be positioned 2 to 3 cm above the clavicle, in the space of the V formed between the sternal and clavicular heads of the sternocleidomastoid. Besides the surface stimulators, a monopolar needle (C) with surface electrode as anode can be used for stimulation. The neck is placed in a neutral or slightly extended position.

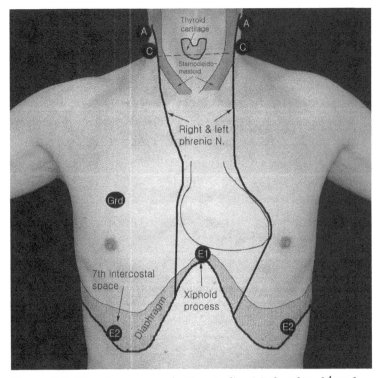

Figure 5-9. *Phrenic nerve conduction studies–Markand et al.[4] and Bolton et al.[5] techniques.*

Reference Values

Markand et al.[4] $N = 50$ Age, 31 to 72 years (mean, 50)

Latency, 9.75 ms = mean $\pm$ 2.5 standard deviation (SD)

Amplitude, >0.4 millivolts (mV)

Bolton et al.[5]

Latency, 6.3 $\pm$ 0.8 ms

Amplitude, 597 $\pm$ 139 microvolts (μV)

Reference electrode (E2) is separated from the E1 electrode by 16 cm.

Distance between stimulation and the E1 electrode is measured.

MacLean et al.[6] $N = 60$ (subject, 30)

Latency, 7.4 $\pm$ 0.6 ms (range, 6.0 to 9.0)

Amplitude, 0.8 $\pm$ 0.4 mV (range, 0.2 to 2)

Needle stimulation

Comments Care must be taken to avoid concurrently stimulating the nearby brachial plexus. Side-to-side comparisons of latency and amplitude are very useful.

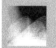

Greater Auricular Sensory Nerve Conduction Studies

(Fig. 5-10)

Recording Electrode Placements

E1 The E1 active electrode is placed on the back of the ear lobe.

E2 The E2 reference electrode is positioned 2 cm distal to the E1 electrode on the back of the ear lobe.

Stimulation

The stimulation is performed antidromically at the lateral border of the sternocleidomastoid muscle, approximately at the midpoint between the mastoid process and the sternum.

---

[4] Markand ON, Kincaid JC, Pourmand RA et al: Electrophysiologic evaluation of diaphragm by transcutaneous phrenic nerve stimulation. *Neurology* 1984;34:604–614.
[5] Bolton CF: AAEM minimonography no. 40: Clinical neurophysiology of the respiratory system. *Muscle & Nerve* 1993;16:809–818.
[6] MacLean IC, Mattioni TA: Phrenic nerve conduction studies: A new technique and its application in quadriplegic patients. *Arch Phys Med Rehabil* 1991;62:70–72.

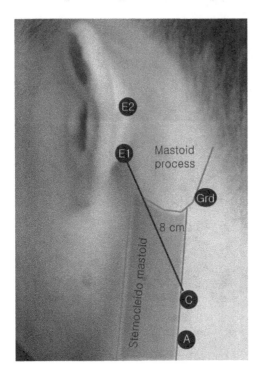

Figure 5-10. *Greater auricular sensory nerve conduction studies.*

Reference Values

Palliyath[7] *N* = 35 Age, 21 to 66 years

Latency (peak) (ms)	Amplitude (μV)	Conduction velocity (m/s)
1.7 ± 0.2	12.7 ± 4.1	46.8 ± 6.6

Distance, 8 cm

Kimura et al.:[8] *N* = 64 Mean age, 45.7 years (14 to 88)

Latency (ms)		Amplitude (μV)
Onset	Peak	
1.3 ± 0.2	1.9 ± 0.2	22.4 ± 8.9

Comments The test may be valuable in differentiating between the pre- and the postganglionic lesions of the second and third cervical roots.

---

[7] Palliyath SK: A technique for studying the greater auricular nerve conduction velocity. *Muscle & Nerve* 1984;7:232–234.

[8] Kimura I, Seiki H, Sasao SI, et al.: The greater auricular nerve conduction study: A technique, normative data and clinical usefulness. *Electromyogr Clin Neurophysiol* 1987;27:39–43.

Spinal Accessory Nerve to the Trapezius Muscle

(Fig. 5-11A, Fig. 5-11B)

Recording Electrode Placements

E1 and E2 A plastic bar electrode is used. The recording electrodes are placed in three different areas of the trapezius: upper trapezius, 5 cm lateral to the C7 spinous process; middle trapezius, midway between the midpoint of the scapular spine and at the same level of the thoracic spinous process; lower trapezius, two fingerbreadths from the spinal column at the level of the scapular lower angle.

Stimulation

Stimulation is performed at the posterior border of the sternocleidomastoid, midway between the mastoid process and the suprasternal notch at the level of the upper margin of the thyroid cartilage.

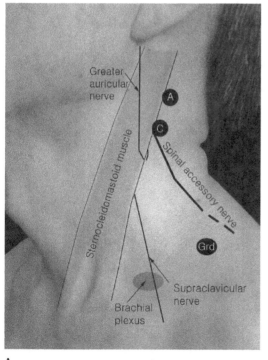

A

Figure 5-11. *A: Spinal accessory nerve stimulation.*

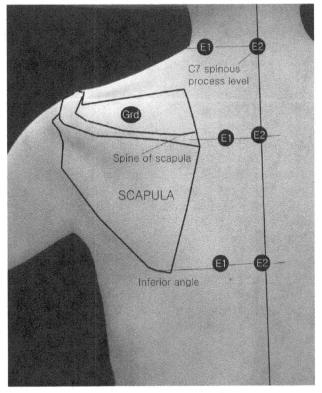

B

Figure 5-11. *(Continued)* **B:** *Spinal accessory nerve conduction studies to the trapezius: upper, middle, and lower.*

Reference Values

Cherrington[9] $N = 25$ Age, 10 to 60 years

Latency to upper trapezius, 1.8 to 3.0 ms

Kraft[10]

Latency, 1.8 to 3.0

Amplitude, 3 to 4 mV

Green and Brien[11] Subject $= 21$ Age, 18 to 65 years

Latency (ms)

to upper trapezius,: 2.1 $\pm$ 0.2 (1.5 to 2.9)

---

[9] Cherington M: Accessory nerve. Conduction studies. *Arch Neurol* 1968;18:708–709.

[10] Kraft GH, Johnson EW: *Proximal nerve conduction and late responses.* American Association of Electromyography and Electrodiagnosis Workshop Boston, Sept. 1986.

[11] Green RF, Brien M: Accessory nerve latency to the middle and lower trapezius. *Arch Phys Med Rehabil* 1985;66:23–24.

to middle trapezius: 3.0 ± 0.2 (2.2 to 3.8)

to lower trapezius: 4.6 ± 0.3 (3.9 to 5.6)

Shanker and Means[12] $N = 16$ Age, 56 to 65

	Upper	middle	lower
Latency (ms)	2.1 ± 0.6	2.7 ± 0.6	5.6 ± 0.8
Amplitude (μV)	1.4 ± 0.5	2.7 ± 1.5	1.2 ± 0.2

Comments This nerve can be affected in situations of radical neck dissection, shoulder girdle neuropathy, space occupying lesions, peripheral neuropathy, etc.

Supraclavicular Sensory Nerve Conduction

(Fig. 5-12)

Recording Electrode Placements

E1 Disposable digital ring electrode of self-adhesive surface strip as the active elctrode is placed over the outer surface of the clavicular shaft.

E2 The same type of the active electrode is placed approximately 3 cm distal to the E1 electrode placement.

Bar electrode with the E1 and E2 electrodes embedded in a plastic bar can also be used.

Stimulation

The cathode is placed at the posterior border of the sternocleidomastoid muscle at the level of the lower margin of the thyroid cartilage.

Reference Values[13] $N = 25$ (50 nerves), Age 36.2 ± 10.8 years (21 to 60 years)

	Latency (ms)		Amplitude (μv)
	Onset	Peak	
Right	1.3 ± 0.2 (0.9 to 1.6)	1.7 ± 0.1 (1.4 to 1.9)	11.5 ± 2.7 (7 to 18)
Left	1.3 ± 0.1 (1.0 to 1.6)	1.7 ± 0.2 (1.3 to 2.0)	10.7 ± 2.7 (6 to 16)

Comments The supraclavicular sensory nerves arise by a common trunk derived from the C3 and C4 roots and are divided into three branches: medial, intermediate, and lateral. The intermediate branch is easily palpated over the midshaft of

---

[12] Shanker K, Means KM: Accessory nerve conduction in neck dissection subjects. *Arch Phys Med Rehabil* 1990;71:403–405.

[13] Lee HJ: Electrophysiologic evaluation of supraclavicular nerves. *Muscle & Nerve* 2004;29:878–879.

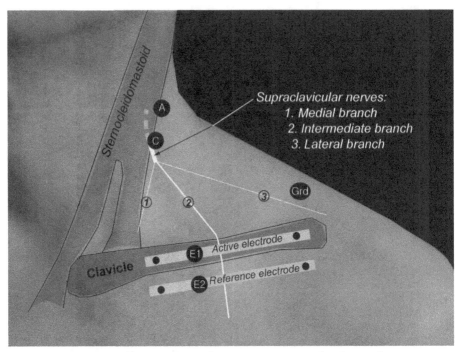

Figure 5-12: *Supraclavicular sensory nerve conduction study.*

the clavicle. To ensure a proper stimulation to the nerve, the cathode may need more superior or inferior repositioning along the posterior border of the sternocleidomastoid muscle. Firm pressure of the stimulator may be helpful, particularly in a patient's neck with large amounts of subcutaneous tissues. The test can be performed either lying supine or in a sitting position in a chair with the chin slightly up. Stimulus intensities usually require no more than 10 milliamperes (mA).

 Abbreviations

cm, centimeter; ms, millisecond; CMAP, compound muscle action potential; SD, standard deviation; mV, millivolt; μV, microvolt; mA, milliamperes.

CHAPTER 6

Short-Segment Incremental Study

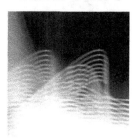

The short-segment incremental stimulation in 1-centimeter (cm) intervals can provide a unique contribution in evaluating the distal segment of the nerves. This technique can be applied in the following nerves:

1. Median motor nerve short-segment incremental study (SSIS) at the wrist. (Fig. 6-1, Fig. 6-2)

2. Ulnar motor nerve SSIS at the wrist.[1,2] (Fig. 6-3, Fig. 6-4, Fig. 6-5)

3. Peroneal motor nerve SSIS at the ankle. (Fig. 6-6, Fig. 6-7)

4. Tibial motor nerve SSIS at the ankle. (Fig. 6-8, Fig. 6-9)

    Reference values (1,2,3,4), ≤0.4 ms/cm

 Abbreviations

cm, centimeter; SSIS, short-segment incremental study.

---

[1] Kimura J: *Electrodiagnosis in diseases of nerve and muscle: Principles and Practice*, 3rd ed. New York: Oxford University Press, 2001.

[2] McIntosh RA, Preston DC, Logigian EL: Short-segment incremental studies to localize ulnar nerve entrapment at the wrist. *Neurology* 1998;50:303–306.

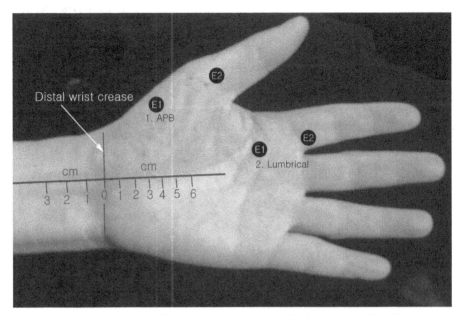

Figure 6-1. *Transcarpal short-segment incremental stimulation of median nerve.*

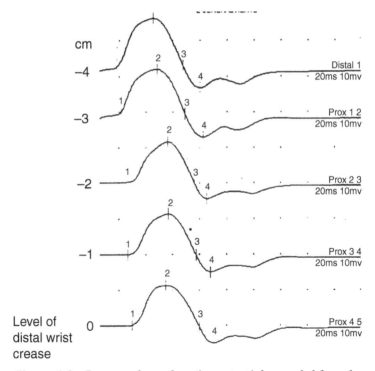

Figure 6-2. *Compound muscle action potentials recorded from the abductor pollicis brevis in transcarpal median nerve short-segment incremental study.*

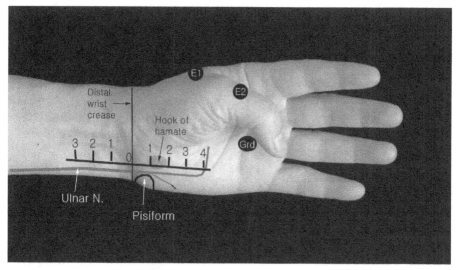

Figure 6-3. *Short-segment incremental study of the ulnar nerve at the wrist.*

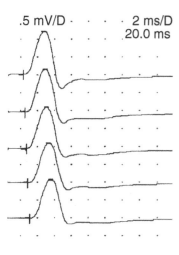

Figure 6-4. *Ulnar motor nerve short-segment incremental study at the wrist (across Guyon's canal).*

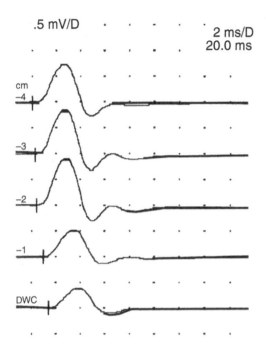

Figure 6-5. *Partial ulnar motor nerve conduction block between 1 and 2 cm distal to the distal wrist crease. Compound muscle action potentials were from the first dorsal interosseus.*

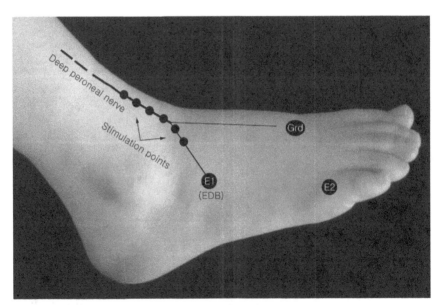

Figure 6-6. *Short-segment incremental study of the deep peroneal nerve.*

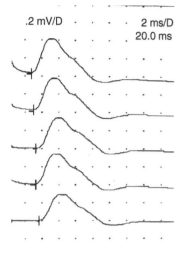

.2 mV/D   2 ms/D
              20.0 ms

Figure 6-7. *Compound muscle action potentials recorded from deep peroneal nerve motor short-segment incremental study at the ankle.*

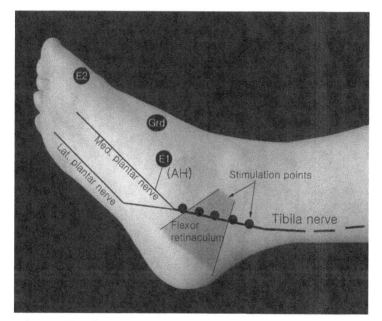

Figure 6-8. *Short-segment incremental study of the tibial nerve at the ankle.*

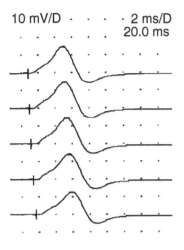

10 mV/D · · · · 2 ms/D
· · · · · · 20.0 ms

Figure 6-9. *Compound muscle action potentials recorded from short-segment incremental study of the tibial nerve across the flexor retinaculum at the ankle.*

CHAPTER 7

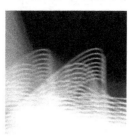

Reflex and Long Latency

 ## Blink Responses

General Electrical stimulation of the supraorbital nerve, a sensory branch of the trigeminal nerve, elicits the blink reflex response, which consists of two separate components: an early R1 and a late R2. Visual and auditory stimuli give a response with only one component. Whereas R1 is evoked only on the side of electrical stimulation, R2 is recorded bilaterally with unilateral electrical stimulation. The patient is either positioned in an armchair, relaxed, and with the eyes half-closed, or placed in a warm room, supine, and with eyes gently closed.

Recording Electrode Placements

E1 The active surface electrode is placed on the belly of the orbicularis oculi below the canthus. To pick up consensual R2 on a second channel, a second pickup (E1) is attached to the opposite orbicularis oculi muscle. A second ground is not needed.

E2 The reference electrode is placed on the side of the nose.

Ground The ground is placed on the forehead or cheek.

Stimulation (Fig. 7-1, Fig. 7-2)
Electrical stimulation is applied over the supraorbital nerve, which is in the groove that is palpable at the medial third of the superior orbit, with the cathode placed over the supraorbital foramen. The infraorbital or mental nerve can be used instead of the supraorbital. Stimulation intensity is usually 3 to

8 milliamperes (mA) (up to 16 to 20 mA), with duration of stimulus between 0.1 and 1 msec. Stimulus of low intensity causes the second response of the blink reflex to have a prolonged latency. Thus, it is necessary to determine the stimulus intensity that will evoke the maximum R2 amplitude. With better stimulus control, there is less variability and more reproducibility of responses.

Electromyograph Settings

Frequency, 8 Hz to 8 kHz

Sweep speed, 5 milliseconds per division (ms per div) (may need 10 ms per div if R2 latency is prolonged)

Sensitivity, 50 to 100 microvolts (μV)/div

Rate, not to be more than 1 per s (a faster rate may produce habituation)

Reference Values $N = 83$ normal adults, supraorbital nerve stimulation

R1 Component Latency 10.6 $\pm$ 2.5 ms [mean + 3 standard deviations (SD)]. It is delayed if it exceeds 13.0 ms. In normal patients, the difference between values for R1 on each side is less than 1.2 ms. Because R1 appears only ipsilaterally, to compare right with left, both sides must be stimulated. Reflex latency is measured from the stimulus artifact to the initial deflection of the evoked potential.

R2 Component Latency Direct R2 (ipsilateral to the side of stimulus) is 31 $\pm$ 10 ms (mean + 3 SD). It is delayed if it exceeds 40 ms. The reflex latency is measured from the stimulus artifact to initial deflection of the potential. Consensual R2 latency (contralateral to the side of stimulus) is 32 $\pm$ 11 ms (mean + 3 SD). It is delayed if it exceeds 41 ms. The difference between values for R2 consensual and R2 direct is normally less than 5 ms (mean + 3 SD). This measurement requires only "one" stimulus, because R2 appears ipsilaterally and contralaterally to the side stimulated.

Amplitude

R1, 0.38 $\pm$ 0.23 millivolt (mV)

R2, 0.53 $\pm$ 0.24 mV

Neonates $N = 30$

R1 component latency, 12.1 $\pm$ 0.96 ms (mean $\pm$ 1 SD)

R2 direct component latency, 35.95 $\pm$ 2.45 ms (mean $\pm$ 1 SD)

The contralateral R1 often is absent. It was bilaterally absent in one-third and usually ipsilateral only in the other two-thirds.

Amplitude

R1, 0.51 $\pm$ 0.18 mV

R2, 0.39 $\pm$ 0.19 mV

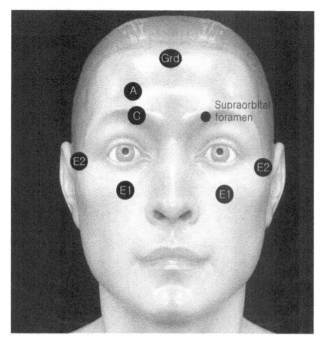

Figure 7-1. *Placement of electrodes and stimulators for blink responses.*

Comments

R1 usually is a biphasaic or triphasic wave (occasionally polyphasic). It tends to habituate slowly and is a brief, relatively synchronous reflex. It is more stable with repeated trials and better suited for assessing nerve conduction of the trigeminal and facial nerves.

R2 is polyphasic and habituates quickly with a decrease in amplitude and duration with repetitive stimulation. R2 correlates with a clinically observed blink of the eyelids.

1. Latency is measured from the stimulus artifact to the initial deflection of the evoked potential (R1 or R1). Kimura[1] suggests using the shortest latency of eight stimulations.

2. Both R1 and R2 waves probably are due to a polysynapatic brain stem reflex, the blink reflex, with the afferent arc provided by the sensory branches of the trigeminal nerve and the efferent arc provided by the facial nerve motor fibers.

R1 is affected by lesions in:
    trigeminal nerve (afferent arc)
    pons (central arc)
    facial nerve (efferent arc)

[1] Kimura J, Powers JM, Van Allen MW: Reflex response of orbicularis oculi muscle to supraorbital nerve stimulation: Study in normal subjects and in peripheral facial paresis. *Arch Neurol* 1969; 21:193–199.

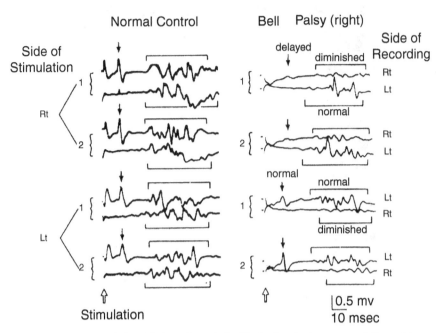

Figure 7-2. *Two right-sided and two left-sided stimulations were delivered in each case to show consistency. In the patient, R1 (arrows) and R2 (single brackets) were delayed and small on the right side and normal on the left side regardless of the side stimulated. This finding indicates a lesion involving the efferent arc of reflex (facial nerve) on the right side. (Kimura et al.[2])*

R2 is affected by:
    level of consciousness
    habituation
    lateral medullary lesion
    contralateral hemispheric lesion
    parkinsonism
    medication [diazepam (Valium)]

3. When the supraorbital nerve is stimulated, both R1 and R2 are regularly elicited in normal patients.

4. When the infraorbital nerve is stimulated, R2 is always present, but R1 is inconsistent in normal patients.

5. When the mental nerve is stimulated, R2 is inconsistent, and R1 is present only rarely in normal patients.

---

[2] Kimura J, Giron LT, Young SM: Electrophysiological study of Bell's palsy. Electrically elicited blink reflex in assessment of prognosis. *Arch Otolaryngol* 1976;102:140–143.

[3] Kimura J, Bodensteiner J, Yamada T: Electrically elicited blink reflex in normal neonates. *Arch Neurol* 1977;34:246–249.

H Reflex Latency to the Gastrocnemius

(Fig. 7-3)

Braddom's Technique[4]

E1 The patient is prone with the feet suspended over the edge of the table or with a pillow placed under the ankle. The E1 active electrode is placed on the bisecting point of a line connecting the popliteal crease and the proximal flare of the medial malleolus.

E2 The reference electrode is attached over the Achilles tendon.

Electromyography Machine Settings

Filters, 8 Hz to 8 kHz

Sweep speed, 5 to 10 ms/div

Sensitivity, 200 to 500 μV/div

Pulse duration, 0.5 to 1.0 ms

Frequency of stimulation, 0.2 Hz

Stimulation

Percutaneous stimulus with low-intensity current (submaximal stimulus) is used. The stimulation pulses of long duration (i.e., 0.5 to 1 ms) are used to preferentially activate a large diameter of sensory fibers. The cathode is proximal and is placed over the tibial nerve in the popliteal fossa at the level of the popliteal crease. The H waves are more easily recorded with the muscle at rest, although contraction of the recording muscle may enhance the H reflexes. Placing an anode over the patella may avoid a large stimulus artifact.

Reference Values

Braddom and Johnson[4] (Fig. 7-4) $N = 125$ Mean age = 39 years (18 to 79)

Predicted H latency (ms): 9.14 + 0.46 × leg length (cm) + 0.1 × age (years).

A difference between two legs of 1.2 ms (3 standard errors) may be considered significant, assuming equal leg lengths.

Tonzola et al.[5]

Technique similar to that of Braddom and Johnson: recording over the soleus

[4] Braddom RL, Johnson EW: Standardization of H reflex and diagnostic use in S1 radiculopathy. *Arch Phys Med Rehabil* 1974;55:161–166.
[5] Tonzola RF, Ackil AA: Shahani BT, et al.: Usefulness of electrophysiological studies in the diagnosis of lumbosacral root disease. *Ann Neurol* 1981;9:305–308.

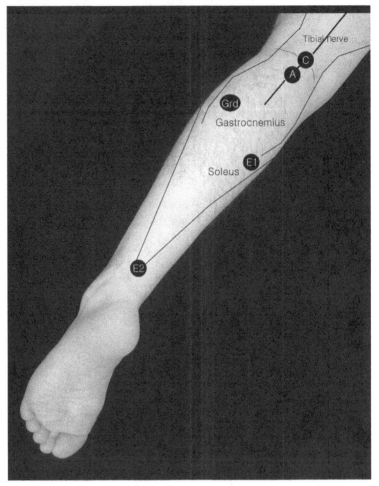

Figure 7-3. *H reflex recording from either soleus or gastrocnemius muscle.*

Height (cm)	H reflex latency (ms)
147 to 160	28.5 ± 1.8
163 to 175	29.9 ± 2.1
178 to 193	31.5 ± 1.2

Latencies more than 2 SDs or absent responses were considered abnormal.

Comments The H wave is thought to be due to the H reflex, a monosynaptic reflex evoked by direct electrical stimulation of large group II afferent fibers. The H wave is recognized as an unchanging muscle-evoked action potential, which occurs at latency of 28 to 35 ms in normals when measured from the gastrocnemius-soleus muscle in adults. It appears at submaximal stimulus either before or shortly after the appearance of the M response. With an increase in stimulus intensity, the maximal H wave can be seen when the M response is submaximal. Further increase in the stimulus intensity increases the amplitude of the M

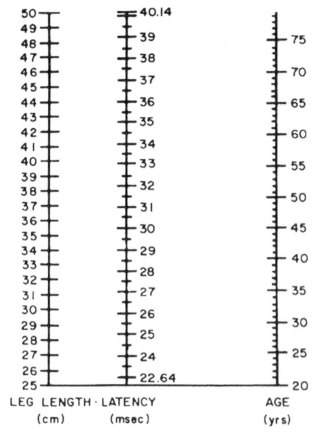

Figure 7-4. *Nomogram of the simultaneous regression of H wave latency on leg length and age. (Braddom and Johnson.[6])*

response and reduces the amplitude of the H wave. At supramaximal stimulus, the H wave disappears and sometimes is replaced by an F wave, but an H wave may be obtained if the stimuli are timed with phasic contractions of the muscles. Johnson[6] suggests measuring latency and comparing it with the predicted value. If latency is prolonged, or clinical history and physical examinations are highly suggestive of radiculopathy, then contralateral latency should be determined. A 1.2-ms or greater difference may be significant. In addition, an abnormal H reflex latency requires evaluation of sensory conduction (e.g., sural nerve) and motor conduction (e.g., tibial or peroneal nerve) to rule out neuropathy. The H wave normally is present at birth, but after the age of 6 months it is present only in the gastrocnemius-soleus and flexor carpi radialis muscles and occasionally can be recorded from the hamstrings and quadriceps muscles. The H wave is triphasic, with an initial positive deflection and a large negative deflection in the gastocnemmius-soleus muscle. The highest amplitude of the H reflex is up

---

[6] Braddom RL, Johnson EW: Standardization of H-reflex and diagnostic use in S1 radiculopathy. *Arch Phys Med Rehabil* 1974;55:161–166.

to 50% to 100% of the maximum M wave. Active contraction of the antagonist muscle can inhibit the H reflex.

Marked shortening or lengthening of the muscle from which the H wave is being recorded can inhibit the reflex. Sleep also may inhibit the reflex. The H wave latency is abnormal in a strictly sensory S-1 radiculopathy. The H wave latency becomes abnormal immediately or shortly after injury to the S-1 nerve root. The H wave latency allows better differentiation between L-5 and S-1 radiculopathy. The H wave may not be present bilaterally in persons over the age of 60 years.

F Wave in the Upper Extremity

(Fig. 7-5)

General The F wave is not a reflex because the afferent and efferent arcs of this response consist of the same α motor axon.

Pickup The active surface electrode for the median nerve is over the abductor pollicis brevis. The active surface for the ulnar nerve is over the abductor digiti quinti. (This placement is the same as standard median or ulnar motor surface nerve placement.)

Reference For the median nerve, the reference is on the distal phalanx of the thumb; for the ulnar nerve, it is on the fifth digit.

Ground The ground is between the stimulation and pickup sites.

Stimulation Stimulation can be applied at the wrist, at the elbow, or in the axilla; however, axillary stimulation is difficult unless the collision technique is used. Exact sites of stimulation are not described. The stimulating electrode is distal and not proximal. Supramaximal stimulation is used.

Electromyograph Settings

- Frequency, 8 Hz to 8 kHz

- Sweep speed, 5 ms/div

- Gain, 250 μV

Distance The distance from the point of stimulus to the seventh cervical spine is measured as follows: Surface measurements are made with the patient in the upright position and the arm abducted 90 degrees. The hand is supinated for the median nerve and pronated for the ulnar nerve. Measurements are made along the course of the nerve to the axilla and then around the back of the shoulder (posteriorly) to the seventh cervical spinous process.

Normal Values[7] ($N = 33$)

---

[7] Kimura J: F-wave velocity in the central segment of the median and ulnar nerves. A study in normal subjects and in the patients with Charcot-Marie-Tooth disease. *Neurology (Minn)* 1974;24:539–546.

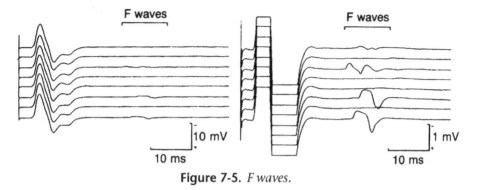

Figure 7-5. *F waves.*

Latency is measured to onset of the F wave and is the minimal latency after several trials (8 to 10 F waves)

Latency values (mean ± 1 SD ms)

Site	Median nerve	Ulnar nerve
Wrist	29.1 ± 2.3	30.5 ± 3.0
Elbow	24.8 ± 2.0	26.0 ± 1.8
Axilla	21.7 ± 2.8	21.9 ± 1.9

Latency difference between two stimulus points (mean ± 1 SD ms)

Site	Median nerve	Ulnar nerve
Elbow-wrist	4.3 ± 0.8	4.1 ± 0.8
Axilla-elbow	3.5 ± 0.5	4.1 ± 0.9

$$\text{F wave velocity (m/s)} = \frac{(\text{distance from stimulus point to C-7 spine}) \times 2 \text{ (mm)}}{(\text{F latency} - \text{M latency}) - 1 \text{ ms}}$$

F wave velocity

Median nerve	m/s (mean ± 1 SD ms)
Wrist-spinal cord	59.2 ± 3.9
Elbow-spinal cord	62.2 ± 5.2
Axilla-spinal cord	64.3 ± 6.4

Ulnar nerve	m/s (mean ± 1 SD ms)
Wrist-spinal cord	56.7 ± 2.9
Elbow-spinal cord	59.4 ± 4.7
Axilla-spinal cord	63.1 ± 5.9

Characteristics of F Wave Versus H Wave and M Wave

1. In contrast with the H wave, the F wave can be recorded from almost every skeletal muscle in the adult. The latency of the F wave is longer, with more distal sites of stimulation.

2. The amplitude of the F wave usually is less than that of the H wave. The F wave often is not present with each stimulus.

3. Supramaximal stimulus, which abolishes the H wave, is used for recording F waves.

4. The F wave has a smaller amplitude than the M wave and is variable in latency and configuration when recorded with surface electrodes.

Comments

1. Latency values are not useful until the exact sites of stimulation are indicated and standards are established.

2. The F wave becomes abnormal immediately after an injury.

3. One cannot distinguish between acute and chronic radiculopathy

4. It receives innervation from multiple nerve roots; hence, it may be normal when only one root is destroyed.

5. F waves do provide a means to measure conduction along the most proximal segment of a nerve.

 ## F Wave in the Lower Extremity

General The F wave is not a reflex because the afferent and efferent arcs of this response consist of the same α motor axon.

PERONEAL NERVE (PATIENT PRONE)

Pickup The active surface electrode is placed over the extensor digitorum brevis muscle in the anterior lateral aspect of the proximal midtarsal level.

Reference The reference is placed on the fifth digit.

Ground The ground is placed between the stimulation and pickup sites.

Stimulation Stimulation can be applied at the ankle, just lateral to the tibialis anterior tendon, or in the popliteal space over the lateral third of the flexor skin crease. The cathode is proximal, and supramaximal stimulation is used.

Electromyograph Settings

- Frequency, 8 Hz to 8 kHz

- Sweep speed, 5 ms/div

- Gain, 200 to 500 μV

Distance The distance is measured from the stimulation site to the lower border of the thoracic-12 spinous process by way of the greater trochanter of the femur.

Normal Values ($N = 66$) The shortest of 10 latencies is taken.

Peroneal nerve F wave latency from ankle, 51.3 $\pm$ 4.7 ms (mean $\pm$ 1 SD)

Peroneal nerve F wave latency from knee, 42.7 $\pm$ 4.0 ms (mean $\pm$ 1 SD)

Peroneal nerve F wave nerve conduction velocity (NCV) (ankle to spinal cord), 53.5 $\pm$ 3.7 ms (mean $\pm$ 1 SD)

Peroneal nerve F wave NCV (knee to spinal cord), 56.3 $\pm$ 4.9 ms (mean $\pm$ 1 SD)

$$F \text{ wave velocity (m/s)} = \frac{(\text{distance from stimulus to T-12}) \times 2 \text{ (mm)}}{(\text{F latency} - \text{M latency}) - 1 \text{ (ms)}}$$

TIBIAL NERVE (PATIENT PRONE)

Pickup The active surface pickup is placed over the abductor hallucis muscle, 1 cm behind and 1 cm below the navicular tubercle.

Reference The reference is placed on the first digit.

Ground The ground is placed between the stimulation and pickup sites.

Stimulation Stimulation can be applied at the ankle, 1 cm posterior to the medial malleolus, or at the knee in the popliteal fossa. The cathode is proximal, and supramaximal stimulation is used.

Distance Distance is measured from the stimulation sites to the lower border of the thoracic-12 spinous process by way of the greater trochanter of the femur.

Electromyograph Settings

Frequency, 8 Hz to 8 kHz

Sweep speed, 5 ms/div

Gain, 200 to 500 μV

Normal Values[8] ($N = 66$) The shortest of 10 latencies is taken.

Tibial nerve F wave latency from ankle, 52.3 $\pm$ 4.3 ms (mean $\pm$ 1 SD)

Tibial nerve F wave latency from knee, 43.5 $\pm$ 3.4 ms (mean $\pm$ 1 SD)

---

[8] Kimura J, Bosch P, Linday GM: F-wave conduction velocity in the central segment of the peroneal and tibial nerves. *Arch Phys Med Rehab* 1975;56:492–497.

Tibial nerve F wave NCV (ankle to spinal cord), 51.3 ± 2.9 ms (mean ± 1 SD)

Tibial nerve F wave NCV (knee to spinal cord), 54.4 ± 3.6 ms (mean ± I SD)

Comment Stimulation usually is tolerated better at the knee than at the ankle.

Sympathetic Skin Response

(Fig. 7-6, Fig. 7-7)

Recording Electrode Placements

Hand The E1 active electrode is placed on palm, 3 cm proximal to the second web space and the E2 reference electrode is placed on the distal phalanx of the third digit.

Foot The E1 electrode is attached on plantar surface, 3 cm proximal to the first web space and the E2 electrode is placed over the second toe.

Ground The electrode is positioned at the wrist or ankle proximal to the recording electrodes.

Electromyography Machine Settings

Filters, 2 Hz (0.5) to 5 kHz (500 to 2,000 Hz)

Sweep speed, 500 ms/div

Sensitivity, 200 μV/div

Pulse duration, 0.2 ms

Stimulus intensity, 15 to 20 mA

Interval of stimulation, one every 15s

Stimulation

Hand recording For recording the sympathetic skin response, the contralateral or same side median nerve is stimulated at the wrist or at the elbow with the cathode proximal.

Foot recording The tibial nerve is stimulated at the ankle with the cathode proximal.

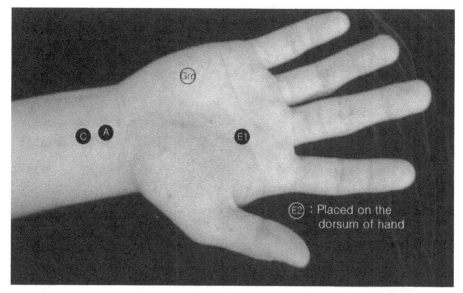

Figure 7-6. *Placement of recording electrodes and stimulators for sympathetic skin responses.*

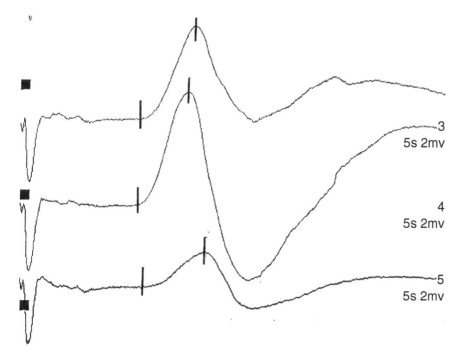

Figure 7-7. *Sympathetic skin response conduction studies with median nerve stimulation and the responses recorded from the hand.*

Reference Values[9] $N = 30$

Recording site	Latency (s)	Amplitude (μV)
Palm	1.52 ± 0.13	479 ± 105
Foot	2.07 ± 1.06	101 ± 40

Comments For testing sympathetic skin response, the room should be quiet with the lights dimmed. Habituation and variability in amplitude or morphology are common with repeated stimulations.

 Abbreviations

mA, milliamperes; Hz, hertz; ms, milliseconds; div, division; μV, microvolts; SD, standard deviation; mV, millivolts; cm, centimeters; NCV, nerve conduction velocity.

---

[9] Knezevic W, Bajada S: Peripheral autonomic surface potential: A quantitative technique for recording sympathetic conduction in man. *J Neurol Sci* 1985; 67:239–251.

Motor Nerve Conduction Studies in Premature Infants, Infants, and Children

CHAPTER 8

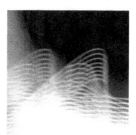

1. The motor nerve conduction velocity (MNCV) values of newborns are about half those of adults.

2. By age 3 years, the MNCV values are in the lower adult range.

3. By age 5 years, the MNCV values are essentially the same as those for adults.

4. Premature infant values (Cerra and Johnson)[1]
    a. Premature ulnar MNCV ($N = 19$), 20.2 ± 2.6 meters per second (m per s); range, 16.5 to 24.6 m per s.
    b. Premature peroneal MNCV ($N = 17$), 19.1 ± 4.2 m per s; range, 13.7 to 28.3 m per s.

5. The MNCV for the median, peroneal, and ulnar nerves for term infants, children, and adolescents are graphed in Figs. 8-1, 8-2, and 8-3. These figures, which express the mean ± 2SD, are derived from the work of Gamestorp.[2]

6. In children, the median and tibial nerves are the most readily accessible for study.

Abbreviations

MNCV, motor nerve conduction velocity; m per s, meters per second; SD, standard deviation.

---

[1] Cerra D, Johnson EW: Motor conduction velocity in premature infants. *Arch Phys Med Rehabil* 1962; 43:160–164.
[2] Gamstorp I: Normal conduction velocity of ulnar, median, and peroneal nerves in infancy, childhood, and adolescence. *Acta Paediatr Scand* 1963;146(Suppl):68–76.

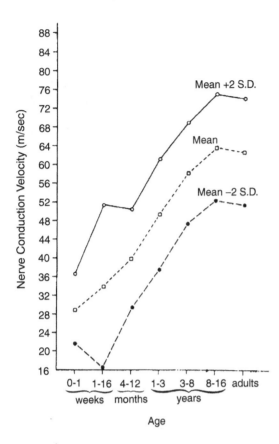

Figure 8-1. *Median motor nerve conduction velocity (mean ± 2SD) for term infants, children, and adolescents. (From DeLisa JA, Lee HJ, Baran EM, et al.:* Manual of nerve conduction velocity and clinical neurophysiology, *3rd ed. New York: Raven Press 1994: 187–189.)*

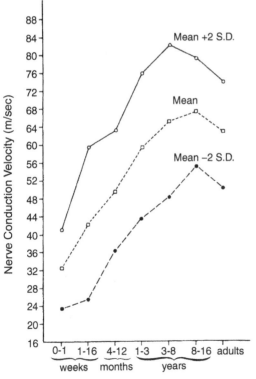

Figure 8-2. *Ulnar motor nerve conduction velocity (mean ± 2SD) for term infants, children, and adolescents. (From DeLisa JA, Lee HJ, Baran EM, et al.:* Manual of nerve conduction velocity and clinical neurophysiology, *3rd ed. New York: Raven Press 1994: 187–189.)*

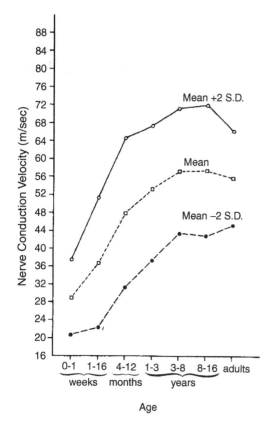

Figure 8-3. *Peroneal motor nerve conduction velocity (mean ± 2SD) for term infants, children, and adolescents. (From DeLisa JA, Lee HJ, Baran EM, et al.:* Manual of nerve conduction velocity and clinical neurophysiology, *3rd ed. New York: Raven Press 1994: 187–189.)*

CHAPTER 9

Repetitive Stimulation (Neuromuscular Junction)

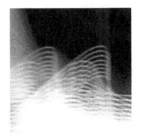

(Fig. 9-1, Fig. 9-2, Fig. 9-3)

Repetitive stimulation techniques can be used in diagnosing diseases of the neuromuscular junction; however, technical errors can give erroneous results, and careful attention to technique is essential.

1. For 24 hours before testing the patient must discontinue any medication that affects the neuromuscular junction.

2. The muscle and joint(s) it crosses are immobilized to minimize movement artifact, and the stimulating and recording electrodes are secured to avoid any movement. Immobilization is best achieved with muscles stretched and joint(s) extended.

3. The skin temperature is maintained at 34°C (94°F) to avoid false-negative results.

4. All stimuli must be supramaximal.

5. In myasthenic syndrome (Lambert-Eaten syndrome), the deficit is present in any muscles tested.

6. If the patient is suspected of having botulism, any clinically weak muscle is tested.

7. In myasthenia gravis, muscle weakness increases with exertion but improves with rest and with anticholinesterase drugs. Proximal muscle testing is much more sensitive than distal muscle testing; however, testing proximal muscles is technically more difficult.

Proximal Stimulation

a. Facial nerve: Stimulate behind the earlobe at the stylomastoid foramen with the active recording electrode over the nasalis muscle.

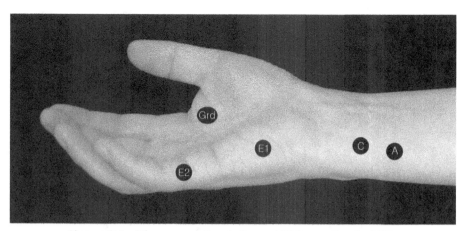

Figure 9-1. *Ulnar nerve stimulation—ADM recording for RNS.*

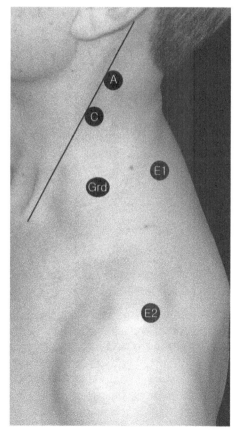

Figure 9-2. *Spinal accessory nerve stimulation—upper trapezius recording.*

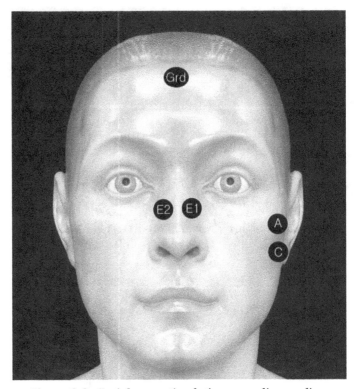

Figure 9-3. *Facial nerve stimulation—nasalis recording.*

b.   Brachial plexus/axillary nerve: Stimulate at Erb's point with the active record-ing electrode over the deltoid muscle. This technique is painful, and move-ment artifact can be a problem.

c.   Musculocutaneous nerve: Stimulate in the axilla with the active electrode over the biceps muscle. With this technique, the stimulus can be unstable.

d.   Femoral nerve: Stimulate in the inguinal region with the active electrode over the vastus medialis muscle. This technique can be painful.

e.   Spinal accessory nerve: Stimulate the nerve as it descends along the posterior border of the sternocleidomastoid muscle with the active electrode over the upper trapezius at the angle of the neck and shoulder. The patient is upright in a chair; the arms are adducted and extended with the hand holding the bottom of the chair. Exercise is obtained by having the patient shrug the shoulders against his/her own resistance.

Distal Stimulation

a.   Ulnar nerve: Most investigators test the ulnar nerve distally. Stimulate the ulnar nerve at the wrist with the active electrode placed over the abductor digiti minimi muscle.

b. Median nerve: Stimulate the median nerve at the wrist with the active electrode over the abductor pollicis brevis muscle. The disadvantage of this technique is that the thumb is difficult to immobilize.

8. During each portion of the test (the single response, the 2 per second(s) stimulation, the 10-s postexercise), the potential amplitude often decreases during the first four responses. Thus, most investigators measure the fifth response, compare its amplitude with that of the first response of the train, and calculate the percentage of change.

9. In a rigidly controlled system, a decrement of the fifth successive potential (compared with the first) by 10% is definitely abnormal in distal muscles. In proximal muscles, where rigid control is more difficult to obtain, only decrements of more than 20% are considered abnormal.

10. The following are important to observe during testing:
    a. Amplitude of the initial response to a single nerve supramaximal stimulation
    b. Presence or absence of a decrement during repetitive stimulation at a slow rate
    c. Presence or absence of a decrement or increment after isometric exercise and then stimulation at a slow rate
    d. Postactivation facilitation
    e. Postactivation exhaustion
    f. Change in response after anticholinesterase drugs

11. Actual technique (Fig. 9-4, Fig. 9-5, Fig. 9-6, Fig. 9-7)

To rule out possible underlying peripheral neuropathy, perform routine motor and sensory nerve conduction studies, preferably in the ulnar and sural nerves. Before applying repetitive stimuli on the ulnar nerve at the wrist,

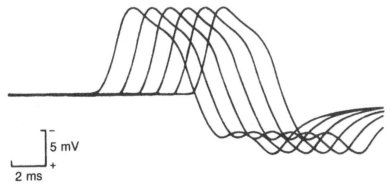

5 mV

2 ms

Figure 9-4. *RNS in a normal person. (From* AAEM glossary of terms in clinical electromyography, *2001, Fig. 13, with permission.)*

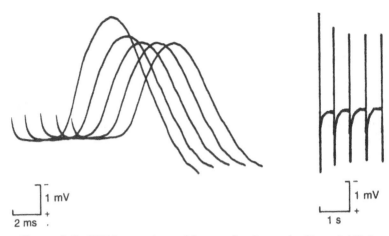

1 mV

2 ms

1 mV

1 s

Figure 9-5. *RNS in a patient with myasthenia gravis. (From* AAEM glossary of terms in clinical electromyography, *2001, Fig. 14, with permission.)*

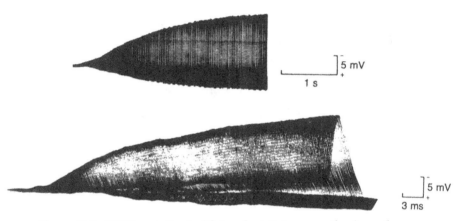

5 mV

1 s

5 mV

3 ms

Figure 9-6. *RNS in a patient with Lambert-Eaton myasthenic syndrome. Repetitive ulnar nerve stimulation at a rate of 50 Hz. (From* AAEM glossary of terms in clinical electromyography, *2001, Fig. 16, with permission.)*

estimate the amount of stimulus intensity and current pulse width for supramaximal stimulation on that nerve. Then, the same intensity with current pulse width is applied in the program (menu) of repetitive stimulation.

a. To obtain the single response: In an unexercised muscle, initially use a high voltage to obtain a supramaximal response; then observe the peak-to-peak amplitude of the initial muscle action potential.

b. Wait 1 min before stimulating at a frequency of 2 Hz or 3 Hz for 3 s, looking for a decrement. For screening purposes, a train of three to five

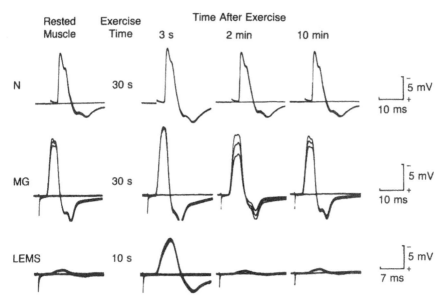

Figure 9-7. *Repetitive nerve stimulations in a normal person (N) and in patients with myasthenia gravis (MG) and Lambert-Eaton myasthenic syndrome (LEMS).* (From AAEM glossary of terms in clinical electromyography, *2001, Fig. 17, with permission.*)

stimuli is adequate. To test reproducibility of the decrement, a muscle must be rested 1 min between tests.

c. Wait at least 1 min (until the amplitude is back to the initial amplitude and use it as the baseline before exercise) before having the patient perform isometric exercises for 10 s (30 s if the muscle is not clinically weak).

d. Ten seconds after the exercise facilitation is completed, start to stimulate at 2 or 3 Hz for 3 s. Repeat this at 30 s, and at 1,2,3, and 5 min to check for postactivation exhaustion or facilitation. (According to the literature, 2 min appears to be the most sensitive time.)

e. Fast rates of stimulation with a 20 to 50 Hz for 10 to 50 s as a form of maximum voluntary contraction if the subject cannot cooperate. This test is useful for detecting an incremental response in myasthenic syndrome or subsequent postactivation exhaustion.

12. Figure 9-4 indicates results seen with repetitive stimulation in normal individuals and in patients with myasthenia gravis, myasthenic syndrome, and botulism.

13. A more sensitive method for evaluating the status of the neuromuscular junction is jitter study of a motor fiber pair by single fiber electromyography. If the repetitive test is abnormal, the single fiber EMG test may not be needed.

14. Each laboratory should establish its approach and technique for evaluating possible dysfunction of the neuromuscular junction. The technique is perfected by performing a number of tests on normal persons.

---

[1] Keesey JC: AAEM minimonograph no. 33 electrodiagnostic approach to defects of neuromuscular transmission. *Muscle & Nerve* 1989;12:613–626.

[2] Botelho SY, Deaterly DF, Austin S, et al.: Evaluation of the electromyogram of patients with myasthenia gravis. *AMA Arch Neurol Psychiatry* 1952;67:441–450.

[3] Harvey AM, Masland RL: A method for the study of neuromuscular transmission in human subjects. *Bull Johns Hopkins Hosp* 1941;68:81–93.

[4] Lambert EH: Diagnostic value of electrical stimulation of motor nerves. *Electroencephalogr Clin Neurophysiol* 1962;14(Suppl 22):9–16.

[5] Oh SJ: *Electromyography: Neuromuscular transmission studies.* Baltimore: Williams & Wilkins, 1988.

[6] Schumm F, Stohr M: Accessory nerve stimulation in the assessment of myasthenia gravis. *Muscle & Nerve* 1984;7:147–151.

[7] Slomic A, Rosenfalck A, Buchthal F: Electrical and mechanical response of normal and myasthenic muscle with particular reference to the staircase phenomenon. *Brain Res* 1968;10:1–78.

[8] *AAEM glossary of terms in clinical electromyography. Section II: Illustrations of selected waveforms Figure 13, 14, 15, and 16.* 2001.

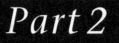

Part 2

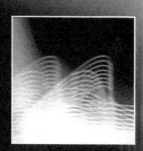

Surface Anatomy for Needle Electro-myography

CHAPTER 10

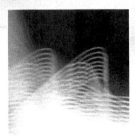

Introduction of Needle Electromyography

A well-planned needle electromyography (EMG) and the patient's cooperation have several advantages. (If you are not sure, consult the experienced electromyographer for the following procedures.)

1. Obtaining the maximal information for the working diagnosis.

2. Minimizing the patient's discomfort.

3. Shortening the length of examination.

4. Minimizing the number of needle penetrations etc.

A complete successful needle electrode examination includes the following:

A. History and physical examination
   1. Review the history for the reasons of referral for the test.
   2. Do a brief physical examination on the focus of the neuromuscular and musculoskeletal system.

B. Take steps to reduce patient anxiety and fear of pain or discomfort
   1. Explain the different phases of the procedure using simple language
   2. Clarify that a disposable needle will be used (except when doing single fiber EMGs)
   3. Explain that no electric current or stimuli will be emitted by the needle
   4. Assure the patient that no substances will be injected through the needle
   5. Inform the patient that sounds will be produced by his or her muscle activity and amplified by the equipment
   6. Reassure the patient that the minimum number of muscles will be tested, consistent with a complete diagnosis

C. Patient position: Find the most comfortable position possible on the examination table or in the chair for the patient and the most convenient position for the examiner.
   1. Supine lying.
   2. Lateral decubitus (side-lying): fetal position (full flexion of neck, trunk, hips, and knees) is very helpful for full relaxation of the paraspinal muscles.
   3. Prone position (to support and relax the testing areas, pillows are placed at various parts of the body: neck, chest, abdomen, hip, knee, (ankle).
   4. Sitting.

Place the patient in a comfortable position on the examination table with the site of needle insertion visible and comfortably reachable for the examiner. The distance from patient to examiner to EMG machine must be comfortably reachable.

D. Preparation of study areas
   1. Expose the area to be studied.
   2. Clean the skin areas to be tested with alcohol and wait for it to evaporate before inserting the needle. Needling a wet area of skin can burn
   3. Cover the unexposed limb or trunk for the patient's comfort if the room is cold.

E. Identification of the muscle to be tested muscle using the landmarks
   1. Origin and insertion of the muscle
   2. Palpation of the muscle belly or tendon movement of activation of the muscle to be tested
   3. Bones
   4. Boundary of the adjacent muscles
   5. Artery and its pulse

It is necessary to be familiar with surface and functional anatomy before insertion of the needle into the muscle. To confirm proper needle placement, the patient may be asked to activate the testing muscle, but this procedure is not possible in patients with severe motor axonal loss. The deep sitting muscles (e.g., tibialis posterior, flexor digitorum profundus, diaphragm, also refer to text) are very difficult to identify.

F. Order of the muscle sampling on needle exam
   1. Proximal to distal.
      The proximal muscles are usually less sensitive than the distal small muscles on needle insertion
   2. The greatest probability of revealing abnormalities and the weakest muscle may be tested first (more abnormal muscle first in anxious patients and children). One exception is that the end stage of the muscle may not provide proper information about the working diagnosis.

    3. Less painful muscle first.

    4. Some patients prefer needle EMG to nerve conduction study (NCS) (especially electricians)

    5. Consult expert for unfamiliar muscle to be tested or prepare well before the exam well with necessary precaution

G. Avoid needle penetration through the following organs if possible

    1. Major vessels (artery and vein)

    2. Excretory glands

    3. Nerves

    4. Tendon

    5. Viscera

    6. Infection site

    7. Ulcer area

    8. Scar

    9. Edema including lymphedema

H. During needle insertion

    1. Hold the needle firmly by the thumb and fingers.

    2. Make the needle insertion site on the skin taut with the thumb and fingers (e.g., biceps or gastrocnemius).

    3. Insert the needle through the skin at a perpendicular angle (large and thick muscle) or sharp angle (thin layer of muscle).
       Insert the needle quickly for less pain!
       Concentric needle—initially insert the needle at a perpendicular angle (direction to the skin or muscle in large muscle but parallel to the muscle fibers—monopolar needle too). Use a sharp angle for thin layer muscle (e.g., facial muscles).
       An extra-long needle (75 mm) is necessary for very obese patients.

    4. Guide the path of needle in the muscle with the fingers so that the needle avoids puncturing the viscera (e.g., serratus anterior, rhomboid, trapezius, orbicularis oculi, etc.).
       Extra caution is necessary near the viscera, muscles in the neck, chest-thoracic wall (pneumothorax), neck, and abdominal wall muscles.

    5. Move the needle a few millimeters (2 to 3) in steps to check insertional/spontaneous activities and to reduce pain.

    6. To look for spontaneous activity, pause a few seconds after each needle movement in the muscle.

    7. To reduce pain, avoid needle insertion if possible in the following areas: endplate region, nerve, tendon, periosteum.

    8. A needle penetration through the skin, subcutaneous tissue, and muscle should include more than five insertions in a straight line depending on the depth (thickness) of the muscle. Withdraw the needle tip by placing it under subcutaneous tissue or skin and reinserting in the opposite direction.

    9. Check needle insertion sites for bleeding, oozing, leakage of edematous fluid, and bruising. Use firm pressure with dried cotton balls or sterile 2 by 2-inch gauge.

I. Special precautions—diseases/problems:
  1. Infection—HIV positive, viral hepatitis, Creutzfeldt–Jacob disease
     * Use a disposable needle.
     * Wear disposable gloves, mask, goggles, and plastic gowns to prevent these transmissible diseases.
     * Avoid touching equipment (e.g., EMG keyboard, needle connector, extension wires, preamplifier) with hands contaminated with blood or body fluid during the test. Clean contaminated equipment with proper disinfectants (refer to the manufacturer's manual).
     * Clean the equipment or items contaminated with blood or body fluid with a proper concentration of bleach.
     * Do tongue and anal sphincter muscle tests last.
  2. Bleeding disorder—hemophilia, anticoagulant therapy, thrombocytopenia
  3. Rheumatic heart disease, valvular heart disease with prosthetic valves—risk of bacterial endocarditis and transient bacteremia
  4. Extreme obesity—it can be difficult to identify the location of the muscles (e.g., most of the chest or thoracic, abdominal wall wall muscles, diaphragm).

To get all the necessary information for the electrophysiologic diagnosis, any available muscles can be chosen for needle examination. Some muscles are more frequently tested than others. Here are examples of the muscles that appeared in the journal *Muscle & Nerve* (as case reports or minimonograph) for the last 10 years, but it does not mean these muscles are more important than other muscles.

Supraspinatus, infraspinatus, pectoralis major, rhomboid, trapezius, deltoid, biceps, triceps—long head and lateral head, pronator trees, flexor carpi radialis, flexor carpi ulnaris, abductor digiti minimi, first dorsal interosseous, abductor pollicis brevis, extensor digitorum communis, extensor carpi ulnaris, extensor indicis, flexor pollicis longus, flexor digitorum superficialis, flexor digitorum profundus (radial side), opponens pollicis, pronator quadratus, serratus anterior, paraspinous muscles—high cervicals and low cervicals, thoracic praspinals, lumbar paraspinals (by L4 and 5), tibialis anterior, gastrocnemius (medial and lateral), vastus medialis, vastus lateralis, tensor fascia lata, semitendinosus, semimembranosus, gluteus maximus, gluteus medius, biceps femoris—short head, tibialis posterior, abductor hallucis brevis, flexor digitorum longus, abductor digiti quinti, extensor hallucis longus, rectus femoris, adductor longus, extensor digitorum brevis, orbicularis oris, masseter, mentalis, orbicularis oculi, tongue, diaphragm, frontalis.

Abbreviation

EMG, electromyography.

References

Capozzoli NJ: Aseptic technique in needle EMG: Common sense and common practice. *Muscle & Nerve* 1996;18:538.

Stevens JC: *AAEM Course D: Practical suggestions for performing the needle electrode examination* 1995, pp. 27–32.

CHAPTER 11

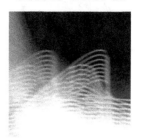

The Hand

Abductor Pollicis Brevis

PATIENT POSITION: Forearm supinated with the palm up.

NEEDLE INSERTION: Insert the needle obliquely from the radial side of the thenar eminence at about the proximal half of the first metacarpal bone.

ACTIVATION: Abduct the thumb with some medial rotation.

CLINICAL NOTES: If inserted too medially in the thenar eminence, the needle will penetrate the flexor pollicis brevis (superficial or deep head); if too deep, opponence pollicis will be penetrated. It is thin and is the most superficial muscle of the thenar muscles. In severe median neuropathy, a needle recording from this muscle may not eliminate the volume-conducted response from adjacent ulnar nerve innervated muscles. This muscle is very painful to needle!

INNERVATION: C8, T1–lower trunk–medial cord–median nerve (recurrent branch).

ORIGIN: Flexor retinaculum, scaphoid, trapezium.

INSERTION: Radial side of the base of the proximal phalanx of thumb, and lateral sesamoid bone of the thumb.

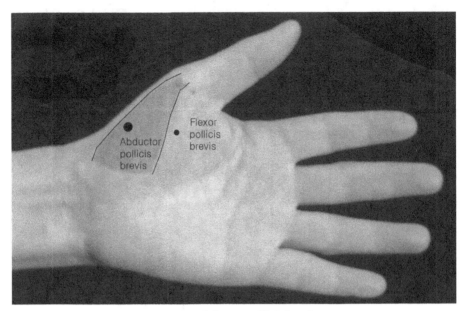

Figure 11-1. *Abductor pollicis brevis.*

 Opponens Pollicis

PATIENT POSITION: Palm up (supination of hand).

NEEDLE INSERTION: This muscle is deep to the abductor pollicis brevis in the thenar eminence. Insert the needle close to the anterior surface of the first metacarpal bone.

ACTIVATION: Opposition of the thumb or flexion of the metacarpal bone of the thumb.

CLINICAL NOTES: It is found deep to the abductor pollicis brevis. It occasionally may be innervated by the deep branch of the ulnar nerve.

INNERVATION: C8, T1–lower trunk–medial cord–median nerve (recurrent branch).

ORIGIN: Flexor retinaculum and trapezium.

INSERTION: Lateral border of the metacarpal bone.

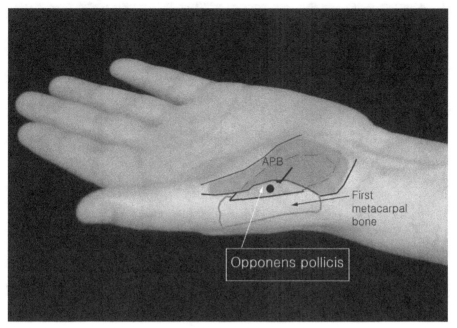

Figure 11-2. *Opponens pollicis.*

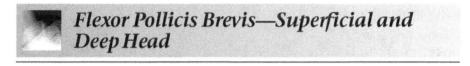

Flexor Pollicis Brevis—Superficial and Deep Head

PATIENT POSITION: Supine with the forearm supinated and palm up.

NEEDLE INSERTION: The thenar eminence can be divided into a lateral half and a medial half by a longitudinal section. Insert the needle into the medial-half area of the thenar eminence.

ACTIVATION: Flex the thumb (proximal phalanx); it also aids opposition and adduction.

CLINICAL NOTES: This muscle is found medial to the abductor pollicis brevis and is somewhat overlapped by it. It is particularly active in a firm grip between the thumb, index, and middle fingers.

INNERVATION: C8, T1–superficial head, median nerve (recurrent branch); deep head, ulnar nerve.

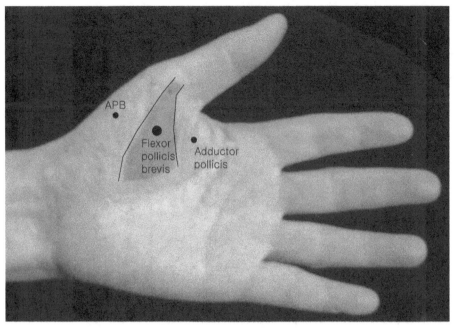

Figure 11-3. *Flexor pollicis brevis—Superficial and deep head.*

ORIGIN: Superficial head; flexor retinaculum, trapezium, and trapezoid. Deep head; trapezoid and capitate.

INSERTION: Radial side of the base of the proximal phalanx of the thumb (medial to the insertion of the abductor pollicis brevis).

 Lumbricals/First Lumbrical

PATIENT POSITION: Palm up (supinated).

NEEDLE INSERTION: Insert the needle at the radial side just proximal to the second metacarpophalangeal joint (MP joint). This site is preferable to the other three lumbricals.

ACTIVATION: Extend the interphalangeal joint of the second, third, fourth, and fifth digits; flex the MP joint.

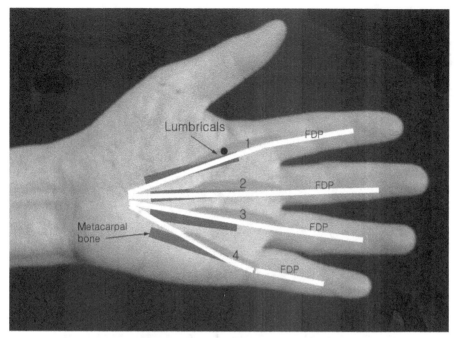

Figure 11-4. *Lumbricals/First lumbrical.*

INNERVATION: The first and second lumbricals are innervated by the median nerve (C8, T1), while the third and fourth are supplied by the deep branch of the ulnar nerve (C8, T1).

CLINICAL NOTES: If the needle is inserted too deeply and proximally on examination of the first lumbrical, it will enter either the adductor pollicis or the first dorsal interosseous.

ORIGIN: Tendons of flexor digitorum profundus.

INSERTION: Lateral margin of dorsal digital expansion at proximal phalangeal level, more distal than the interossei.

First Dorsal Interosseous

PATIENT POSITION: Forearm and hand halfway between supination and pronation.

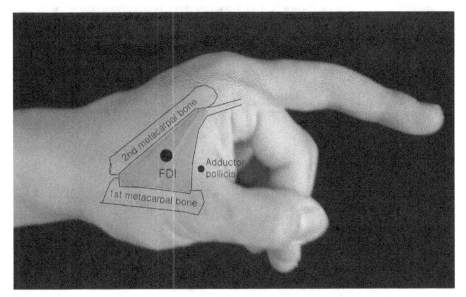

A

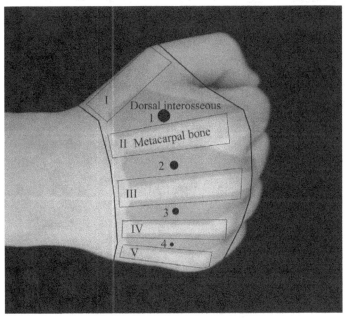

B

Figure 11-5. *First dorsal interosseous.*

NEEDLE INSERTION: Insert the needle at the center (most prominent belly of this muscle) of the dorsal first web space. If inserted too deeply, it will be in the adductor pollicis.

ACTIVATION: Abduct the second digit.

INNERVATION: C8, T1–lower trunk–anterior division–medial cord–ulnar nerve (deep branch)

ORIGIN Lateral head—from the dorsal surface of the proximal half of the ulnar border of the first metacarpal bone.

Medial head—dorsal surface of the radial border of the second metacarpal bone

INSERTION: Radial side of the proximal phalanx of the second digit.

 Adductor Pollicis

PATIENT POSITION: Hand and forearm in the midhalf position.

NEEDLE INSERTION: Insert the needle at the distal half of the ulnar border of the first metacarpal bone obliquely toward the palm and the second meta-carpal bone.

ACTIVATION: Adduct the thumb.

CLINICAL NOTES: If the needle is advanced too medially, it will be in the first dorsal interosseous. It lies deep in the palm in contact with the metacarpals and the interossei muscles.

INNERVATION: C8, T1–lower trunk–anterior division–medial cord–ulnar nerve (deep branch).

ORIGIN: The second and third metacarpal bone, capitate bone, and tendon of the flexor carpi radialis.

INSERTION: Medial side of the base of the proximal phalanx of the thumb and medial sesamoid bone of the thumb.

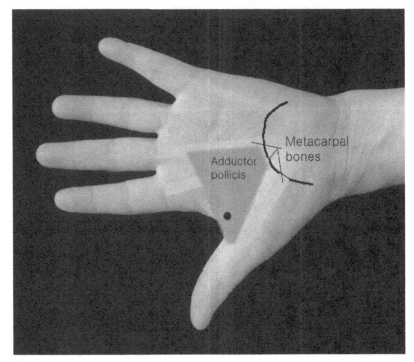

A

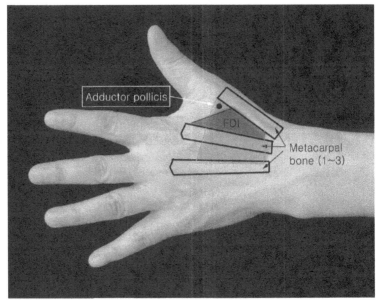

B

Figure 11-6. *Abductor pollicis.*

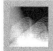

Second Palmar Interosseous

PATIENT POSITION: Palm up.

NEEDLE INSERTION: Insert the needle at the ulnar side of the midhalf of the second metacarpal bone.

ACTIVATION: Adduct the second digit to the third digit.

INNERVATION: C8, T1–lower trunk–medial cord–ulnar nerve (deep branch).

ORIGIN: Entire ulnar side of the palmar surface of the second metacarpal bone.

INSERTION: Same side of the digital expansion of the index finger.
Base of the proximal phalanx of the index finger.

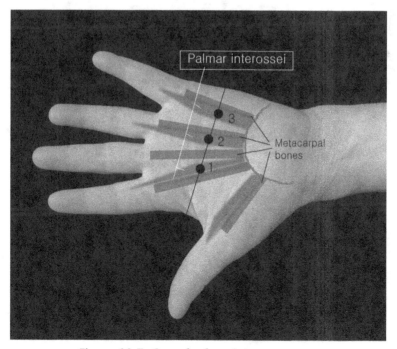

Figure 11-7. *Second palmar interosseous.*

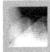 *Abductor Digiti Minimi*

PATIENT POSITION: Forearm supinated with palm up or forearm pronated with palm down.

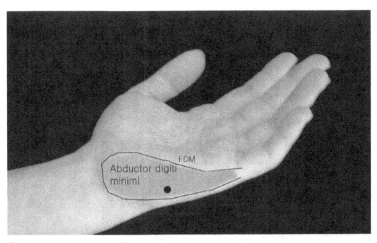

A

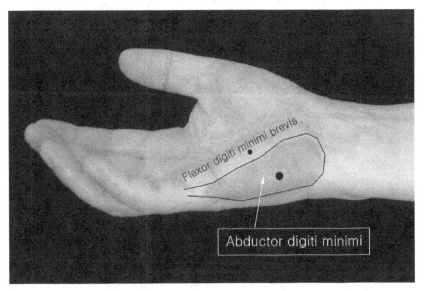

B

Figure 11-8. *Abductor digiti minimi.*

NEEDLE INSERTION: Insert the needle from the ulnar aspect of the hand at about the proximal one-third point between the distal wrist crease and the proximal digital crease.

ACTIVATION: Abduct the little finger away from the ring finger, with flexion of the proximal phalanx at the MP joint.

INNERVATION: C8, T1–lower trunk–medial cord–ulnar nerve (deep branch).

ORIGIN: Pisiform bone and tendon of flexor carpi ulnaris.

INSERTION: Ulnar (medial) side of the base of the proximal phalanx of the fifth digit.

Flexor Digiti Minimi Brevis

PATIENT POSITION: Supine with palm up.

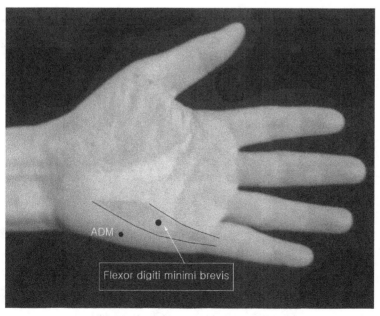

Figure 11-9. *Flexor digiti minimi brevis.*

NEEDLE INSERTION: Insert the needle at the midpoint between the proximal digital crease of the little finger and the distal wrist crease.

ACTIVATION: Flex the little finger at the MP joint.

CLINICAL NOTES: The muscle lies on the radial side of the abductor digiti minimi and may be missing. It is the most superficial of the hypothenar muscles.

INNERVATION: C8, T1–lower trunk–medial cord–ulnar nerve (deep branch).

ORIGIN: Hook of the hamate bone and the palmar surface of the flexor retinaculum.

INSERTION: Ulnar side of the base of the proximal phalanx of the fifth digit.

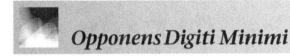

Opponens Digiti Minimi

PATIENT POSITION: Supine with the forearm supinated and palm up.

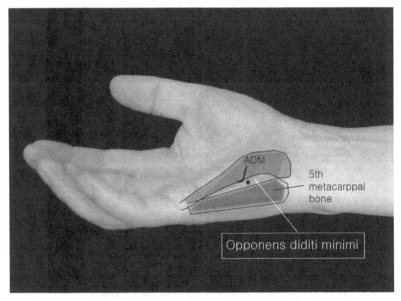

Figure 11-10. *Opponens digiti minimi.*

NEEDLE INSERTION: This muscle lies deep the abductor digiti minimi (ADM) and partly covers the fifth metacarpal bone in the volar aspect of the palm.

Insert the needle at the midhalf of the fifth metacarpal bone from the ulnar side. The needle is inserted close to the bone on the palm side and it advanced radially in the coronal plane. While advancing, the ADM is pushed radially.

ACTIVATION: Opposition of the little finger to the thumb.

INNERVATION: C8, T1–lower trunk–medial cord–ulnar nerve.

ORIGIN: Hook of hamate and flexor retinaculum.

INSERTION: Entire length of the ulnar margin of the fifth metacarpal bone.

 Abbreviations

Mp, metacarpophalangeal; ADM, abductor digiti minimi

CHAPTER 12

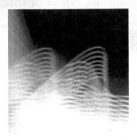

The Forearm

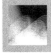 *Pronator Teres*

PATIENT POSITION: Supine with the forearm supinated.

NEEDLE INSERTION: Place the index finger on the cubital fossa and insert the needle medially to the finger at approximately 5 centimeters (cm) below the elbow crease.

ACTIVATION: Pronate the forearm with the elbow slightly flexed.

CLINICAL NOTES: If inserted too deeply, the needle may penetrate the median nerve or brachial artery; too medially, the flexor carpi radialis.

INNERVATION: C6,C7–upper and middle trunk–anterior division–lateral cord–median nerve.

ORIGIN: Medial epicondyle of the humerus and coronoid process of the ulnar.

INSERTION: Lateral surface of the radius to the midline (wraps around the radius).

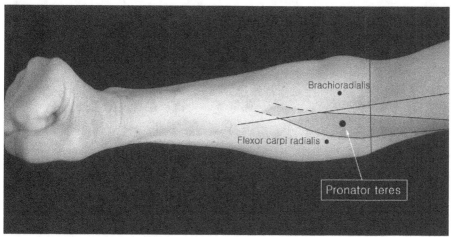

A

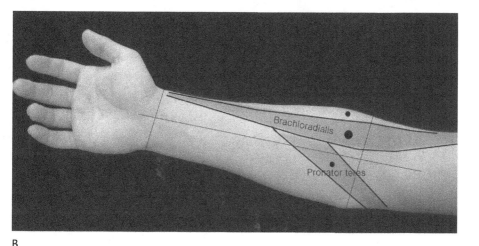

B

Figure 12-1. *Pronator teres.*

Flexor Carpi Radialis

PATIENT POSITION: Supine with forearm supinated.

NEEDLE INSERTION: Insert the needle at the proximal one-third to one-half between the tendon of flexor carpi radialis at the wrist and the medial supracondylar area of humerus. It is medial to the pronator teres. This muscle is medial to the pronator teres. It is a superficial muscle and is not clearly demarcated from the adjacent muscles.

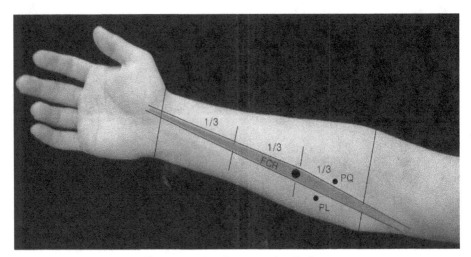

Figure 12-2. *Flexor carpi radialus.*

ACTIVATION: Flex and abduct the wrist (radial deviation).

CLINICAL NOTES: This muscle may be involved in pronator syndrome. If the needle is inserted too laterally, it will be in the pronator teres; if too medially, it will be either in the palmaris longus; if too deeply, it will be in the flexor digitorum superficialis or flexor digitorum profundus.

INNERVATION: C6,C7–median nerve.

ORIGIN: Medial epicondyle of the humerus by a common flexor tendon.

INSERTION: Base of the volar surface of the second metacarpal bone.

 Palmaris Longus

PATIENT POSITION: Supine with forearm fully supinated.

NEEDLE INSERTION: Insert the needle at the proximal one-third of a line drawn between the palmaris longus tendon at the wrist crease and medial epicondyle.

ACTIVATION: Flex the wrist.

CLINICAL NOTES: The muscle is superficial, slender, fusiform, and medial to the flexor carpi radialis. If inserted too deeply, it will be in the flexor digitorum

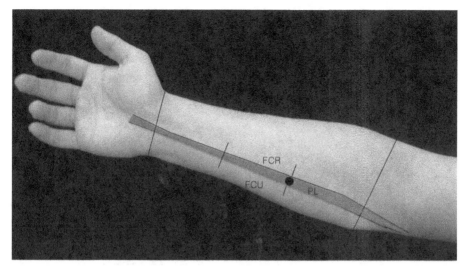

Figure 12-3. *Palmaris longus.*

superficialis. This muscle is absent in 10% to 13% of the population and is subject to a lot of variation.

INNERVATION: C7,C8–median nerve.

ORIGIN: Medial epicondyle of the humerus by a common tendon.

INSERTION: Palmar aponeurosis and flexor retinaculum.

Flexor Digitorum Superficialis (Sublimis)

PATIENT POSITION: Supine with forearm supinated.

NEEDLE INSERTION: Identify the tendons of palmaris longus and flexor carpi ulnaris at the wrist and follow proximally to the midforearm where the needle is inserted. The muscle is more superficial at this point.

ACTIVATION: Flex the middle phalanx of each of the medial four digits.

CLINICAL NOTES: If the needle is inserted too deeply, it will be in the flexor digitorum profundus. Entrapment of the anterior interosseous nerve occurs by either a fibrous origin of this muscle or a tendinous origin of it to the third digit.

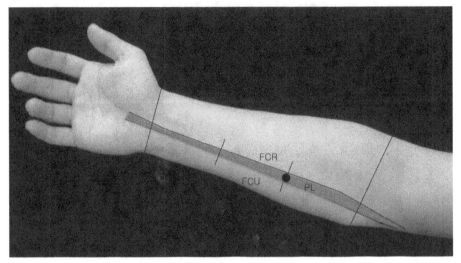

Figure 12-4. *Flexor digitorum superficialis (sublimis).*

INNERVATION: C7,C8 and T1–median nerve.

ORIGIN: Medial epicondyle of the humerus by a common flexor tendon, coronoid process of the ulna, and ulnar collateral ligament of the elbow joint.

INSERTION: Palmar aspect of the middle phalanx of the medial four digits.

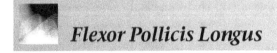

Flexor Pollicis Longus

PATIENT POSITION: Supine with forearm supinated.

NEEDLE INSERTION: Insert the needle at the junction of middle and distal third of the forearm between the brachioradialis and flexor carpi radialis. Before inserting, note the radial pulse at the insertion site.

ACTIVATION: Flex the distal phalanx of the thumb.

CLINICAL NOTES: In diagnostic workup of carpal tunnel syndrome, this muscle is examined to rule out possible more proximal involvement of the median nerve.

INNERVATION: C8, T1–lower trunk–medial cord–anterior interosseous branch (nerve) of the median nerve.

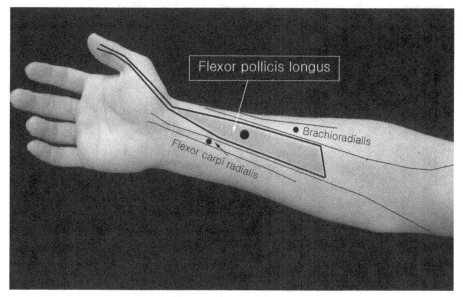

Figure 12-5. *Flexor pollicis longus.*

ORIGIN: Anterior surface of the middle half of the radius, adjoining the anterior interosseous membrane.

INSERTION: Base of the volar surface of the distal phalanx of the thumb.

Pronator Quadratus

PATIENT POSITION: Supine with forearm supinated or pronated.

NEEDLE INSERTION

1. From the ulnar (medial) side of the forearm, insert the needle close to the anterior surface of the ulna, 2 to 3 cm proximal to the ulnar styloid. On insertion, put a finger under the tendon of flexor carpi ulnaris and push it to the radial side.

2. Identify a cleft between the layers of extensor tendons over the dorsal aspect of the distal forearm (distal fourth between the lateral epicondyle and ulnar styloid). Insert the needle between tendons and supinate forearm into a neutral position; slowly advance it through the interosseous membrane and finally into the pronator quadratus.[1]

---

[1] Wertsch JJ: AAEM case report no. 25: Anterior interosseous nerve syndrome. *Muscle & Nerve* 1992;15:977–983.

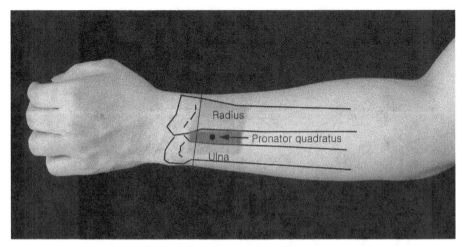

Figure 12-6. *Pronator quadratus.*

CLINICAL NOTES: This is the most distal muscle innervated by the anterior interosseous nerve, examined for conduction study of the anterior interosseous nerve. This is one of the deepest muscles of the forearm flexor muscles.

INNERVATION: C8,T1–lower trunk–medial cord–median nerve–anterior interosseous nerve.

ORIGIN: Anteromedial aspect, distal quarter of the ulna.

INSERTION: Anteromedial, distal quarter of the radius.

 Flexor Carpi Ulnaris

PATIENT POSITION: Supine and forearm supinated.

NEEDLE INSERTION: Insert the needle at the midthird of a line drawn between the ulnar styloid and medial epicondyle. When supinated, this muscle is most medially located. If the needle is inserted too deeply, it will pass into the flexor digitorum sublimis or profundus.

ACTIVATION

1. Flex and abduct (ulnar deviation) the wrist or simply flex and abduct the fifth digit.

2. Abduct the fifth digit without wrist flexion.[2]

---

[2] Roberts MM, Wertsch JJ, Park TA, Mazur A, Oswald TA: Selective activation of the flexor carpi ulnaris. *Muscle & Nerve* 1994;17:1099.

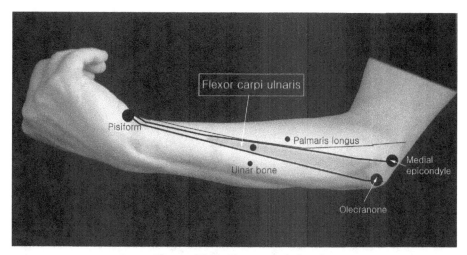

Figure 12-7. *Flexor carpi ulnaris.*

CLINICAL NOTES: In ulnar nerve compression at the elbow, this muscle is often spared.

INNERVATION: C8,T1–lower trunk–medial cord–ulnar nerve.

ORIGIN: Medial epicondyle of the humerus and olecranon.

INSERTION: First into the pisiform bone, then to the hook of the hamate, and finally into the base of the fifth metacarpals by the pisohamate and pisometacarpal ligaments.

Flexor Digitorum Profundus

PATIENT POSITION: Supine with elbow flexed and forearm fully pronated.

NEEDLE INSERTION: Insert the needle from the medial border at the middle third of the ulna and advance it tangentially toward the radial side, pushing the muscle belly of the flexor carpi ulnaris/flexor digitorum superficialis radially.

CLINICAL NOTES: This muscle has a dual innervation—radial side by the median nerve and ulnar side by the ulnar nerve. This is true in about 60% of the cases. In the other 40%, the median and ulnar nerve distributions are 3:1 and 1:3 equally. Examine to verify the selective involvement of the anterior interosseous nerve.

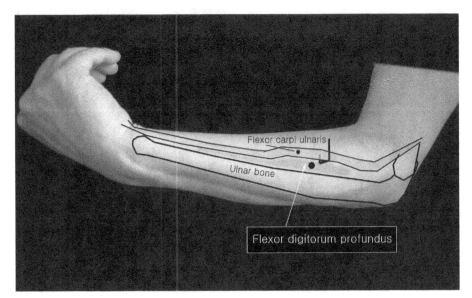

Figure 12-8. *Flexor digitorum profundus.*

Needle placement to this muscle is not easy anatomically or technically. Preferably use the other muscles such as the flexor pollicis longus or pronator quadratus.

INNERVATION: C7, C8, T1–middle and lower trunk–anterior division–median and ulnar nerve.

ORIGIN: Proximal three-fourths of the anterior surface of ulna, medial half of the anterior interosseous membrane, and deep fascia.

INSERTION: Palmar surface of the distal phalanx of each of the medial four digits.

 Brachioradialis

PATIENT POSITION: Supine with forearm supinated.

NEEDLE INSERTION: Identify the cubital fossa by placing the index finger at the elbow. The border of the fossa is formed by the brachioradialis laterally and pronator teres medially. Insert the needle at about 1 cm laterally from the cubital fossa and 1 cm below to the elbow crease with the forearm supinated.

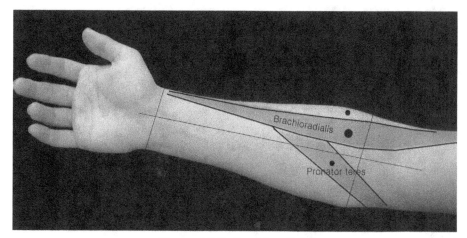

Figure 12-9. *Brachioradialis.*

ACTIVATION: Flex the elbow.

CLINICAL NOTES: Radial neuropathy in the midhumerus or spiral groove usually shows abnormal electromyography findings in the brachioradialis with the triceps spared. Therefore, this muscle is important to identify the localization of radial nerve lesion in a wrist drop.

INNERVATION: C5,C6–upper trunk–posterior devision–posterior cord– radial nerve.

ORIGIN: Lateral supracondylar ridge of the humerus.

INSERTION: Lateral aspect of the radial styloid process.

Extensor Carpi Radialis Longus and Brevis

PATIENT POSITION: Supine with the forearm pronated.

NEEDLE INSERTION

Longus: With the forearm fully pronated, the most prominent area radially just below the elbow is formed by this muscle. Insert the needle 2 to 3 cm distal to the elbow joint over the most prominent area of that muscle bulk.

Brevis: Insert the needle a little bit distal and just lateral to the extensor carpi radialis longus.

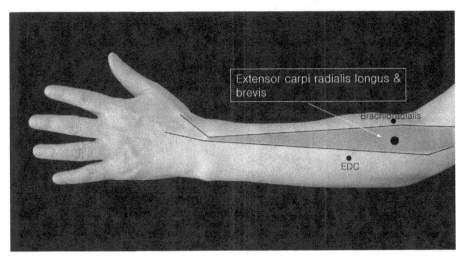

Figure 12-10. *Extensor carpi radialis longus and brevis.*

ACTIVATION: Extend and abduct the wrist, flex the elbow.

CLINICAL NOTES: After innervating the extensor carpi radialis brevis, the radial nerve becomes the posterior interosseous nerve that passes through the supi- nator.

INNERVATION: C6,C7–upper and middle trunk–posterior division– posterior cord–radial nerve.

ORIGIN: Distal third of the lateral supracondylar ridge of the humerus.

INSERTION: Dorsal surface, base of the second metacarpal bone.

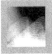 *Extensor Carpi Ulnaris*

PATIENT POSITION: Supine with the forearm pronated.

NEEDLE INSERTION: Insert the needle at the midpoint between the lateral epicondyle and the ulnar styloid.

ACTIVATION: Extend and adduct the hand or abduct and extend the fifth digit.

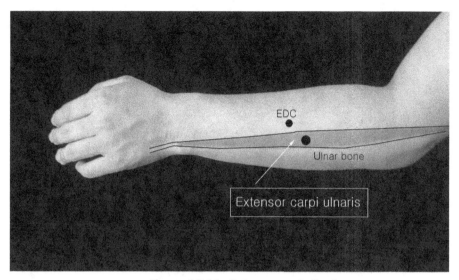

Figure 12-11. *Extensor carpi ulnaris.*

INNERVATION: C7,C8–middle and lower trunk–posterior division–posterior cord–radial nerve (posterior interosseous nerve).

ORIGIN: Lateral epicondyle of the humerus by a common extensor tendon and posterior aspect of the ulna.

INSERTION: Dorsal surface of the base of the fifth metacarpal bone.

 Extensor Digitorum Communis

PATIENT POSITION: Supine with the forearm pronated.

NEEDLE INSERTION: Insert the needle at the upper third in a line drawn between the lateral epicondyle and the midpoint of bilateral styloid at the wrist.

ACTIVATION: Extend the second and third digits.

CLINICAL NOTES: This muscle is examined for single fiber electromyography. This muscle occupies much of the extensor surface of the forearm.

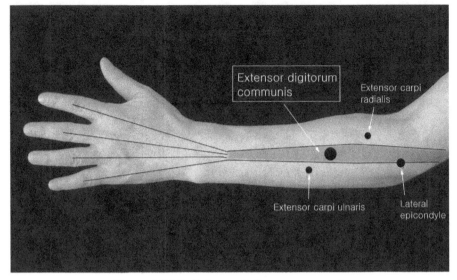

Figure 12-12. *Extensor digitorum communis.*

INNERVATION: C7,C8–middle and lower trunk–posterior division–posterior cord–posterior interosseous nerve (radial nerve).

ORIGIN: Lateral epicondyle of humerus by a common extensor tendon.

INSERTION: Divides into four tendons above the wrist and inserts into the extensor tendon hood with a central slip to the middle phalanx of 2, 3, 4, 5 and two collateral slips to the terminal phalanx of 2, 3, 4, 5.

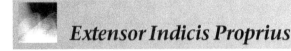

Extensor Indicis Proprius

PATIENT POSITION: Supine with the forearm pronated.

NEEDLE INSERTION: Insert the needle into the distal fourth of the forearm immediately lateral to the radial side of the ulna between the tendons of extensor carpi ulnaris and extensor digitorum. Note this muscle contraction at the distal forearm or wrist may be seen or palpable by extending and flexing the index finger.

ACTIVATION: Extend the index finger.

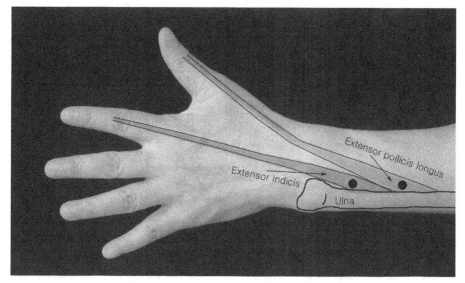

Figure 12-13. *Extensor indicis proprius.*

CLINICAL NOTES: This is the most distally located muscle innervated by the radial nerve and the most distal of the forearm extensor muscles. The muscle can be used in an evaluation of radial nerve conduction. If inserted more proximally, the needle will be in the extensor pollicis longus.

INNERVATION: C7,C8–posterior cord–posterior interosseous nerve (radial nerve).

ORIGIN: Posterior surface of the ulna below extensor pollicis longus and the posterior interosseous membrane.

INSERTION: Head of second metacarpal bone, joins with extensor digitorum tendon to the second finger.

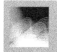

Extensor Pollicis Longus

PATIENT POSITION: Supine with the forearm pronated.

NEEDLE INSERTION: Insert the needle at the middle third of the forearm along the radial side of the ulna.

ACTIVATION: Extend the thumb (distal phalanx).

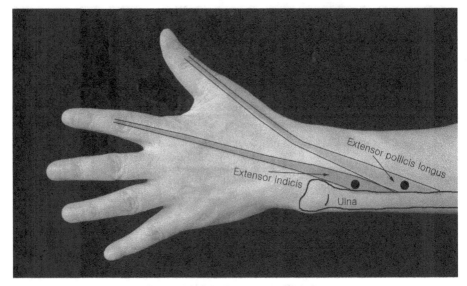

Figure 12-14. *Extensor pollicis longus.*

INNERVATION: C7,C8–middle and lower trunk–posterior division–posterior cord–radial nerve (posterior interosseous nerve).

ORIGIN: Posterior surface of the middle third of the ulna shaft and posterior interosseous membrane.

INSERTION: Dorsal surface of the base of the distal phalanx of the thumb.

Supinator

PATIENT POSITION: Supine with the forearm pronated.

NEEDLE INSERTION: Insert the needle over the radius between the extensor carpi radialis and extensor digitorum communis at the upper third of the forearm.

ACTIVATION: Supinate the forearm.

CLINICAL NOTES: When the deep branch of the radial nerve emerges from the supinator, it is referred to as the posterior interosseous nerve. This muscle may or may not be involved in the posterior interosseous syndrome, although it is not involved in supinator syndrome.

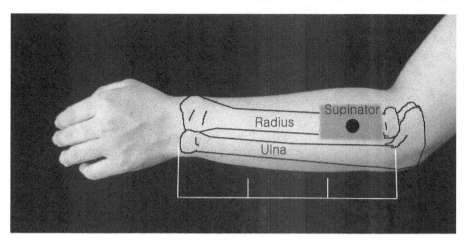

Figure 12-15. *Supinator.*

INNERVATION: C5,C6–upper trunk–posterior division–posterior cord–radial nerve (posterior interosseous nerve).

ORIGIN:

Humeral head (superficial head): Lateral epicondyle of the humerus, radial collateral ligaments of the elbow joint, and annular ligament of the superior radioulnar joint.

Ulnar head (deep head): distal to the radial notch on the posterolateral surface of the ulna or the supinator fossa and crest of the ulna.

INSERTION: Humeral head–lateral surface of the radius.

Ulnar head encircles the radius and inserts into the proximal third of the radius.

 Abbreviation

cm, centimeter.

CHAPTER 13

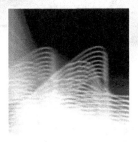

The Arm

 Biceps Brachii

PATIENT POSITION: Supine with the forearm supinated.

NEEDLE INSERTION: Insert the needle just below the midpoint between the shoulder and elbow joint. If needle is inserted too deeply, it will be in the brachialis.

ACTIVATION: Flex the elbow with forearm fully supinated and with external rotation of the arm.

INNERVATION: C5,C6–upper trunk–lateral cord–musculocutaneous nerve.

ORIGIN

Short Head: coracoid process of the scapula, lateral to the tendon of the coraco-brachialis.

Long Head: Supraglenoid tubercle of the scapula.

INSERTION: Radial tuberosity and the lacertus fibrosis (forearm fascia) into the ulnar side of the forearm.

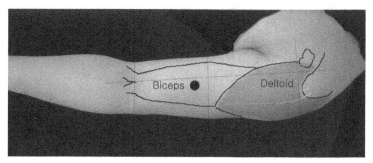

Figure 13-1. *Biceps brachii.*

 Brachialis

PATIENT POSITION: Supine with the arm at the side of the thorax, elbow slightly flexed, and the forearm pronated.

NEEDLE INSERTION: Note the biceps and brachioradialis at the lower one-third of the arm. At the space between the biceps and brachioradialis of the lower one-third of the arm, the needle is inserted toward the front of humerus.

ACTIVATION: Flex the elbow.

CLINICAL NOTES: Similar to biceps brachii. Some of the lateral portion of this muscle may be innervated by the radial nerve.

INNERVATION: C5,C6–upper trunk–lateral cord–musculocutaneous nerve.

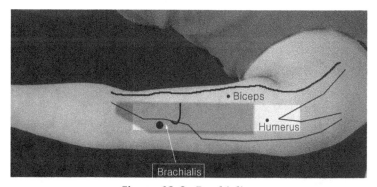

Figure 13-2. *Brachialis.*

ORIGIN: Distal half of the anterior humerus, at the insertion of deltoid.

INSERTION: Ulnar tuberosity and coronoid process of the ulna.

Coracobrachialis

PATIENT POSITION: Supine.

NEEDLE INSERTION: Insert the needle near the junction between the proximal end of the anterior axillary fold (anterior wall) and the anterior border of the deltoid muscle. If the needle is inserted too laterally, it will be in the biceps brachii.

ACTIVATION: Flex, adduct, and externally rotate the arm with elbow flexed.

CLINICAL NOTES: The musculocutaneous nerve pierces this muscle and may become entrapped. Persistence of the lower head of this muscle is associated with the ligament of Struthers, which attaches a supratrochlear spur (from the

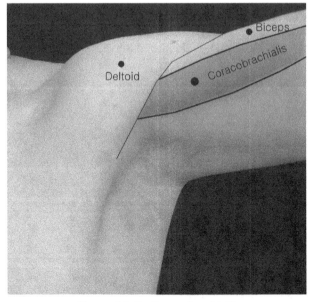

Figure 13-3. *Coracobrachialis.*

anteromedial aspect of the lower humerus) to the medial epicondyle of the humerus and may entrap the median nerve.

INNERVATION: C5, C6–upper trunk–lateral cord–musculocutaneous nerve.

ORIGIN: Coracoid process of the scapula, in common with the tendon of the short head of the biceps.

INSERTION: Anteromedial surface of the midhumerus.

 Triceps

PATIENT POSITION: Lateral decubitus, supine or prone.

NEEDLE INSERTION

1. Long head: Arm abducted at 90 degrees with the elbow extended. At approximately 5 centimeters distal to the posterior axillary fold and posterior to the posterior deltoid, grasp the muscle belly and insert the needle. The posterior axillary fold is formed by the subscapularis, teres major, and latissimus dorsi.

2. Medial head: Arm internally rotated and the forearm extended. Insert the needle about 5 centimeters straight above the olecranon.

3. Lateral head: Insert the needle just posterior to the deltoid tubercle at the midpoint of the arm.

ACTIVATION: Extend the forearm at the elbow.

CLINICAL NOTES: Wrist drop is common, resulting from radial nerve compression in the spiral groove. A needle electromyograph of all three heads and the anconeus are usually normal. Order of recruitment is the medial first, then the lateral, and finally the long head as increased power is needed.

INNERVATION: C6, C7, C8–middle and lower trunk–posterior division–radial nerve.

ORIGIN

Long Head: Infraglenoid tuberosity of the scapula.

Lateral Head: Posterior surgical neck of the humerus above the spiral groove.

Medial Head: Posteromedial half of the humerus below the spiral groove.

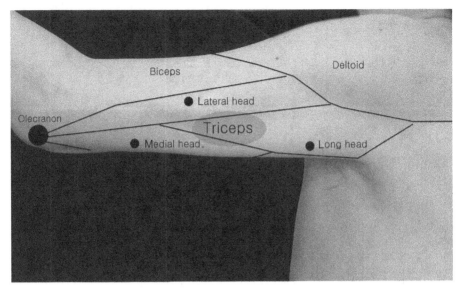

Figure 13-4. *Triceps.*

INSERTION: Proximal end of the olecranon process of the ulna.

Anconeus

PATIENT POSITION: Supine with the elbow flexed and forearm pronated.

NEEDLE INSERTION: Identify the lateral epicondyle, olecranon, and proximal ulna.

Insert the needle about 1 centimeter distal to the lateral epicondyle and advance it toward the medial border of the ulna.

ACTIVATION: Extend the elbow.

CLINICAL NOTES: This muscle is very thin, is triangular, and is located on the back of the elbow joint. In wrist drop with radial neuropathy in the spiral groove of the humerus, this muscle is usually normal. It is innervated by a branch of the radial nerve that leaves the nerve trunk before entering the spiral groove.

INNERVATION: C7,C8–posterior cord–radial nerve.

ORIGIN: Distal part of the back of the lateral epicondyle of the humerus.

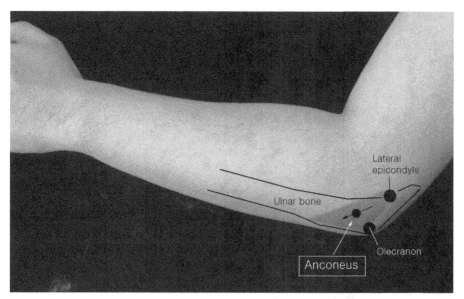

Figure 13-5. *Anconeus.*

INSERTION: Upper fourth of the posterior surface of the ulnar shaft.

Deltoid

PATIENT POSITION: Supine, lateral decubitus, or sitting with the arm at the side.

NEEDLE INSERTION: Insert the needle at the midpoint between the humeral tubercle and deltoid tuberosity. Three parts (anterior, lateral, and posterior) can be examined with separate needling.

ACTIVATION

Abduct the arm (middle deltoid).

Flex the arm (anterior deltoid).

Extend the arm (posterior deltoid).

CLINICAL NOTES: The muscle may also show abnormal electromyograph findings with repeated previous injections. Activation of the deltoid is greatest between 90 and 180 degrees of elevation.

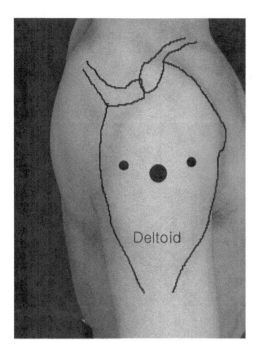

Figure 13-6. *Deltoid.*

INNERVATION: C5, C6–Upper trunk–posterior cord–axillary nerve.

ORIGIN: Anterior aspect of the lateral third of the clavicle, lateral border of the acromion, crest of the scapular spine.

INSERTION: Deltoid tuberosity of the humerus.

CHAPTER 14

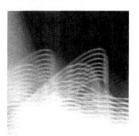

The Shoulder

Supraspinatus

PATIENT POSITION: Lateral decubitus, prone, or sitting.

NEEDLE INSERTION: The supraspinatus fossa is palpable between the medial half of the spine of the scapula and upper trapezius. The needle is inserted into the fossa until it reaches the bone and then is withdrawn slightly. The needle should pass through the trapezius to reach the supraspinatus in the scapular spinous fossa.

ACTIVATION: Abduct the arm at the shoulder.

INNERVATION: C5,C6–upper trunk–suprascapular nerve.

ORIGIN: Medial two-thirds of the supraspinous fossa of the scapula.

INSERTION: Greater tubercle of the humerus.

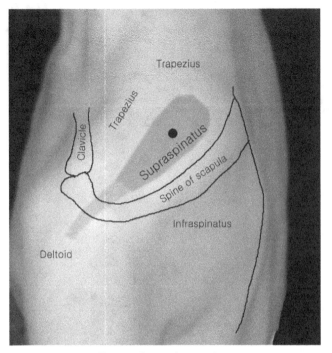

Figure 14-1. *Supraspinatus.*

 Infraspinatus

PATIENT POSITION: Lateral decubitus, prone or sitting.

NEEDLE INSERTION: Note the spine, medial and lateral border of scapula. Insert the needle 2 to 3 centimeters below the scapular spine in the lateral half of the scapula. If the needle is inserted close to the medial border, it must pass through the lower trapezius to reach the infraspinatus.

ACTIVATION: Externally rotate the arm with the forearm flexed.

INNERVATION: C5, C6–upper trunk–suprascapular nerve.

ORIGIN: Medial two-thirds of the infraspinous fossa of the scapula.

INSERTION: Greater tubercle of the humerus.

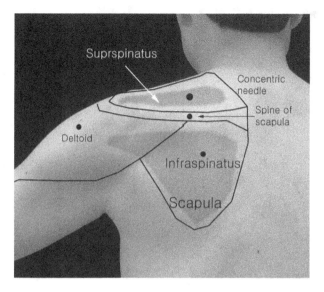

Figure 14-2. *Infraspinatus.*

 Teres Major

PATIENT POSITION: Lateral decubitus or prone.

NEEDLE INSERTION: Note the lateral border and lower angle of scapula, proximal humerus, and posterior axillary fold. Grasp the posterior axillary fold by thumb and index fingers at its lower third, insert the needle at the space between these two fingers, and advance it toward the lateral border of the scapula.

ACTIVATION: Extend, adduct, and internally rotate the arm. Forearm is flexed while moving the hand toward ipsilateral buttock.

INNERVATION: C5,C6–upper trunk–posterior cord–subscapular nerve.

ORIGIN: Dorsal inferior angle (lower third of the lateral border) of the scapula.

INSERTION: Medial lip of the bicipital groove of the humerus, posterior to the tendon of the latissimus dorsi.

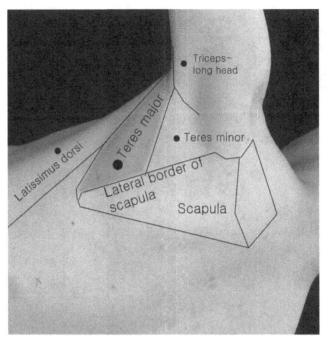

Figure 14-3. *Teres major.*

Teres Minor

PATIENT POSITION: Lateral decubitus or prone.

NEEDLE INSERTION: Note the lateral border of the scapula and proximal humerus. Insert the needle at the upper third of the scapula, just off its lateral border.

CLINICAL NOTES: The muscle is small, short, and narrow, and it is attached to the lateral border of the scapula. It is invested by the fascia of the infraspinatus and sometimes is inseparable from the muscle. The long head of the triceps passes under this muscle at the axilla, and the teres major passes just lateral to the muscle. The teres minor and infraspinatus are occasionally fused. Technically, it is not easy to needle this muscle.

ACTIVATION: External rotation of the arm with the forearm flexed.

INNERVATION: C5,C6–upper trunk–posterior cord–axillary nerve.

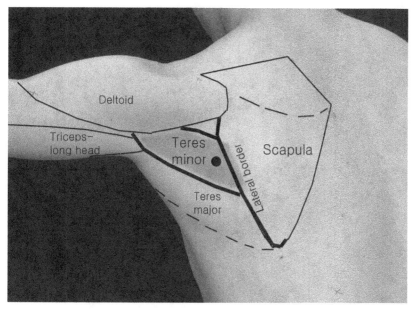

Figure 14-4. *Teres minor.*

ORIGIN: Upper two-thirds of the dorsal surface of the lateral border of scapula.

INSERTION: Greater tubercle of humerus, below the insertion of the infraspinatus.

 Rhomboid Major

PATIENT POSITION: Lateral decubitus or prone.

NEEDLE INSERTION: Identify the lower medial border (just above lower angle) of the scapula and the ribs at the corresponding level of the spinous processes of T2-5. Insert the needle close to the lower medial border of the scapula with care.

ACTIVATION: Arm is placed along the side of the body, elbow flexed, and forearm placed behind back. Ask the patient to elevate the medial border and adduct the scapula toward the vertebrae.

CLINICAL NOTES: This muscle is located deep to the trapezius. It is believed that the findings in this muscle are comparable with those of corresponding

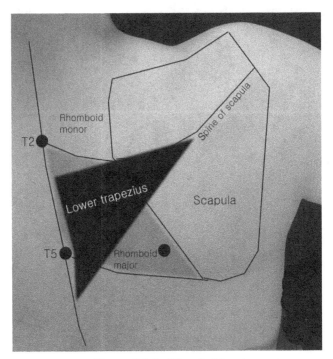

Figure 14-5. *Rhomboid major.*

paraspinal muscles because of direct nerve supply of C5. The muscle examination requires great technical experience and care to avoid a pneumothorax.

INNERVATION: C5 (occasionally from C4)–dorsal scapular nerve.

ORIGIN: Thoracic vertebral spinous processes two through five.

INSERTION: Medial border between the triangular surface at the root of the scapular spine and the inferior angle of the scapula.

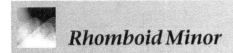

Rhomboid Minor

PATIENT POSITION: Prone or side lying.

NEEDLE INSERTION: Halfway (more closer to the scapula) between the C7 spine and medial end (base) of the spine of the scapula.

ACTIVATION: Retract and elevate the scapula.

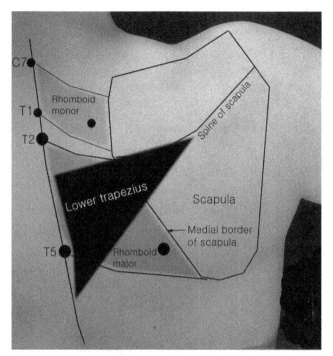

Figure 14-6. *Rhomboid minor.*

CLINICAL NOTES: The muscle is deep to the trapezius.

INNERVATION: C5–dorsal scapular nerve–may also have C4.

ORIGIN: Lower part of ligamentum nuchae, and vertebral spinous processes C7 and T1 vertebrae.

INSERTION: Medial border at the base (end) of the scapular spine.

 Pectoralis Major

CLAVICULAR HEAD (UPPER)

PATIENT POSITION: Supine.

NEEDLE INSERTION: With the arm at 90 degree flexion and external rotation, the muscle bulk can be palpated on the anterior aspect to the deltopectoral groove. Insert the needle at the muscle belly with activation.

ACTIVATION: Adduct, flex, and internally rotate the shoulder (arm).

CLINICAL NOTES: Congenital absence of this muscle has been reported, and the surrounding muscles (e.g., deltoid and coracobrachialis) can compensate for the shoulder motion in the absence of this muscle.

INNERVATION: C5,C6–upper trunk–lateral cord–lateral pectoral nerve.

ORIGIN: Medial two-thirds of the clavicle.

INSERTION: Lateral lip of intertubercular sulcus of humerus.

PECTORALIS MAJOR: STERNAL HEAD (LOWER)

PATIENT POSITION: Supine.

NEEDLE INSERTION: Grasp the anterior axillary fold by the thumb and index finger, and insert the needle at the midportion of the anterior axillary fold.

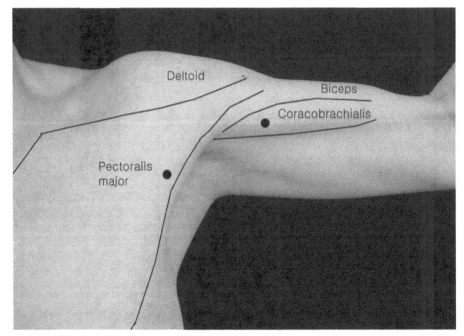

Figure 14-7. *Pectoralis major.*

ACTIVATION: Adduct and internally rotate the arm at the shoulder. The palm of hand is placed over the ipsilateral lower chest wall and some pressure is applied to the chest wall to activate the muscle.

INNERVATION: C7,C8, T1 (sternal part)–middle and lower trunk–medial cord–medial pectoral nerve.

ORIGIN: Sternum and upper six costal cartilages.

INSERTION: Intertubercular sulcus of the humerus.

 Trapezius

PATIENT POSITION: Side lying, sitting, or supine.

NEEDLE INSERTION: The trapezius consists of three parts: upper, middle, and lower.
Preferably examine the upper trapezius. At the angle of the neck, grasp the anterior and posterior parts of the muscle belly, and insert the needle and advance it with care.

ACTIVATION: Raise the patient's shoulder toward his/her upper extremity placed along the side of the body.

CLINICAL NOTES: It is the most superficial of the back muscles, and it is thin. In paralysis of the trapezius, one sees lateral winging of the scapula as it is displaced upward and laterally.

• Tested for accessory neuropathy.

• Pneumothorax may result with misdirection of the needle.

INNERVATION: C3, C4 (cervical plexus)–but is generally believed to be sensory, and accessory nerve (cranial XI).

ORIGIN (O) AND INSERTION (I)

Upper trapezius: (O) External occipital tuberance and medial third of the superior nuchae line and cervical vertebral spinous process, 7.

(I) Lateral one-third of clavicle and acromium.

Middle trapezius: (O) Spinous process of C7 and upper thoracic vertebrae, 1 to 5.

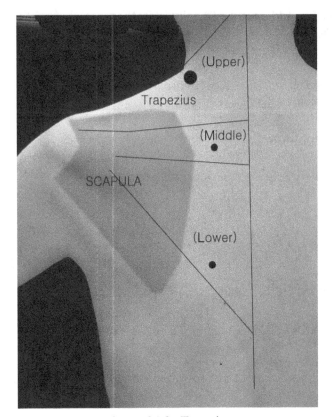

Figure 14-8. *Trapezius.*

(I) Superior lip of the scapular spine.

Lower trapezius: (O) Spinous process of thoracic vertebrae, 6 to 12.

(I) Base of the scapular spine.

 Latissimus Dorsi

PATIENT POSITION: Lateral decubitus or prone.

NEEDLE INSERTION: With arm abducted, flexed, and externally rotated at the shoulder, this muscle can be identified in the posterior axillary fold. At 5 to 10 centimeters distal to the axilla, grasp the posterior axillary fold by two fingers and insert the needle more anteriorly (posteriorly; teres major).

ACTIVATION: Adduct, extend and internally rotate the humerus against resistance.

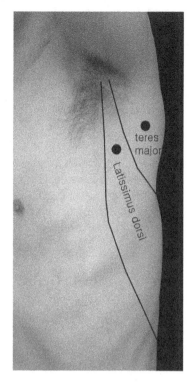

Figure 14-9. *Latissimus dorsi.*

CLINICAL NOTES: Large, triangular, flat muscle that lies in the lower part of the back. It makes up the largest component of the posterior axillary fold. Be cautious to prevent pneumothorax. The teres major may be penetrated if the needle is inserted too close to the lateral border of the scapula.

INNERVATION: C6, C7, C8–posterior cord–thoracodorsal nerve.

ORIGIN: Lower six thoracic vertebral spinous processes, all the lumbar vertebral spinous and transverse processes, sacral spinous processes, and posterior portion of the iliac crest.

INSERTION: Medial lip of bicipital groove of the humerus.

Serratus Anterior

PATIENT POSITION: lateral decubitus or supine with arm flexed.

NEEDLE INSERTION: Anatomic landmarks–anterior axillary line, 5th to 8th ribs anteriorly. Choose one of the above ribs near the anterior axillary line, and place two fingers at the adjacent intercostal spaces. Insert the needle into the muscle over the rib at the space between two fingers and advance it with caution, using two fingers to guide the needle.

ACTIVATION: Ask the patient to push his/her shoulder forward, drawing the medial border of the scapula anteriorly close to the chest wall. Alternatively, ask the patient to flex the arm at 90 degrees with the elbow extended and push forward against the side of a wall or the examiner's hand.

CLINICAL NOTES: Large, curved, quadrilateral-shaped muscle that passes around the thorax. In paralysis of the serratus anterior, one will see medial winging of the scapula. Besides the rhomboid muscle, this is the other muscle innervated directly by C5, C6, and C7 spinal root. Its nerve is the first to arise from the spinal roots, and thus it is very important to test it in brachial plexus, versus root avulsion injuries.

INNERVATION: C5, C6, C7 roots–long thoracic nerve.

ORIGIN: Outer surface and superior border of ribs 1 to 10.

INSERTION: Costal surface of the scapula along the inferior angle and the entire anterior surface of the medial border of the scapula.

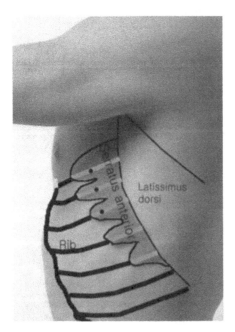

Figure 14-10. *Serratus anterior.*

CHAPTER 15

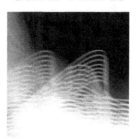

The Foot

 ## Abductor Hallucis

PATIENT POSITION: Supine with the foot supinated.

NEEDLE INSERTION: Insert the needle at the medial side of the sole, just inferior to the navicular bone, and advance it toward the lateral border of the foot.

ACTIVATION: Abduct and flex the big toe. Ask the patient to curl or fan his/her toes.

CLINICAL NOTES: Findings of isolated denervation due to repeated local trauma are common. Interpretation of clinical significance is controversial.

INNERVATION: L5, S1–sciatic nerve–tibial nerve–medial plantar nerve.

ORIGIN: Posterior medial tuberal process of the calcaneus, the flexor retinaculum, and the plantar aponeurosis.

INSERTION: Medial side of the flexor plantar surface of the base of the proximal phalanx of the big toe.

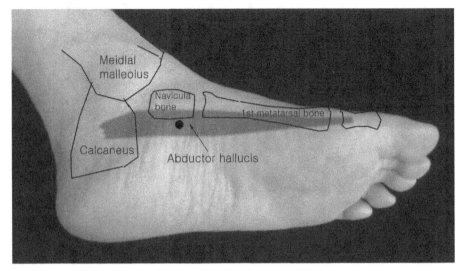

Figure 15-1. *Abductor hallucis.*

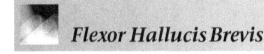

Flexor Hallucis Brevis

PATIENT POSITION: Supine with ankle supinated.

NEEDLE INSERTION: Insert the needle close to the first metatarsal bone medially and advance it to the lateral side of foot.

ACTIVATION: Flex the big toe.

INNERVATION: L5, S1–tibial nerve–medial plantar nerve.

ORIGIN: Cuneiform bones and divides into two bellies.

INSERTION

Medial belly: medial side of the base of the proximal phalanx of the first digit and blends with the abductor hallucis.

Lateral belly: lateral side of the base of the proximal phalanx of the first digit and blends with the adductor hallucis.

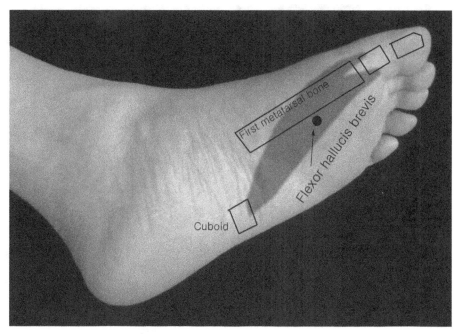

Figure 15-2. *Flexor hallucis brevis.*

 Flexor Digitorum Brevis

PATIENT POSITION: Supine with the foot supinated.

NEEDLE INSERTION: Insert the needle just lateral to the abductor hallucis at the level of the navicular bone and about 1 centimeter off the distal part of the heel pad.

ACTIVATION: Flex the middle phalanges.

CLINICAL NOTES: This muscle is located deep to the plantar aponeurosis and lateral to the abductor hallucis. This muscle is equivalent to the flexor digitorum superficialis in the upper extremity. The lateral plantar nerves and vessels run deep to this muscle toward the lateral part of the foot.

INNERVATION: S2, S3–sacral plexus–sciatic nerve–tibial nerve–medial plantar nerve.

ORIGIN: Medial tubercle of the calcaneus.

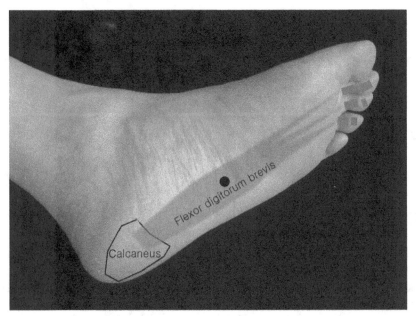

Figure 15-3. *Flexor digitorum brevis.*

INSERTION: Sides of the base of the middle phalanx of the lateral four digits (2,3,4,5).

 Abductor Digiti Minimi

PATIENT POSITION: Side lying, or supine with the foot pronated.

NEEDLE INSERTION: Just inferior to the lateral border of the cuneiform bone of the foot. Or, insert the needle in the space between the distal part of the calcaneus and proximal part of the fifth metatarsal bone.

ACTIVATION: Ask the subject to flex and fan his/her lateral toes. Also, ask the patient to make a cup of his/her foot.

INNERVATION: S1, S2–sciatic nerve–tibial nerve–lateral plantar nerve.

ORIGIN: Lateral tubercle of the calcaneus.

INSERTION: Lateral side of the base of the proximal phalanx of the fifth toe.

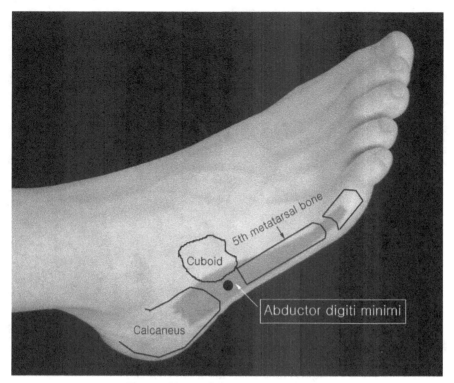

Figure 15-4. *Abductor digiti minimi.*

 First Dorsal Interosseous

PATIENT POSITION: Supine.

NEEDLE INSERTION: Midportion of the first web space (space between first and second metatarsal bones).

ACTIVATION: Abduct the toes (fan toes out).

INNERVATION: S1, S2–sciatic nerve–tibial nerve–lateral plantar nerve.

ORIGIN: Adjacent sides of the first and second metatarsal bones.

INSERTION: Medial side of the base of the proximal phalanx of the second toe.

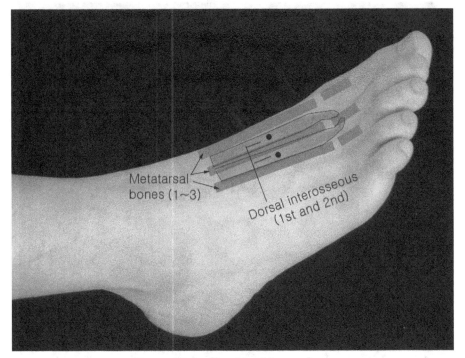

Figure 15-5. *First dorsal interosseous.*

 Extensor Digitorum Brevis

PATIENT POSITION: Supine.

NEEDLE INSERTION: Insert the needle at the proximal one-third of the top of the foot between the tip of the lateral malleolus and the third or fourth toe.

ACTIVATION: Extend the phalanges of the second, third, and fourth toes.

INNERVATION: L5, S1–sciatic nerve–common peroneal nerve–deep peroneal nerve.

CLINICAL NOTES: Superficial, very thin muscle. Insert the needle at a sharp angle (20 to 30 degrees) to the skin. Denervation limited to this muscle due to repeated trauma is common. In about 28% of cases, the lateral portion of this muscle is innervated by the accessory peroneal nerve, which is a branch of the superficial peroneal nerve.

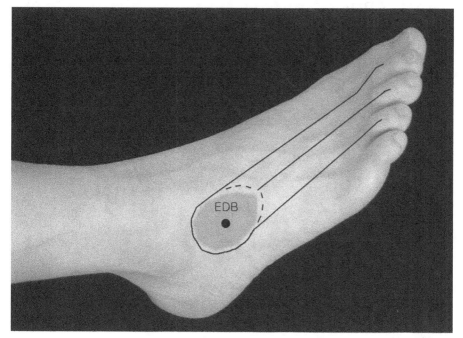

Figure 15-6. *Extensor digitorum brevis.*

ORIGIN: Superolateral surface of the calcaneus, extensor retinaculum, lateral talocalcaneal ligament.

INSERTION: Lateral sides of the tendon of the extensor digitorum longus of the second, third, and fourth toes. Also into the dorsal surface of the base of the proximal phalanx of the great toe.

CHAPTER 16

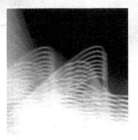

The Leg

 ## *Tibialis Anterior*

PATIENT POSITION: Supine.

NEEDLE INSERTION: Insert the needle approximately 1.5 centimeters lateral to the tibial crest and at the junction of the upper and middle third of the leg.

ACTIVATION: Dorsiflex the ankle and invert the foot.

CLINICAL NOTES: Tibialis anterior tendon is the most prominent and most medial of the dorsal three tendons.

INNERVATION: L4, L5, (S1)–peroneal portion of sciatic nerve–common peroneal nerve–deep peroneal nerve.

ORIGIN: Lateral condyle of tibia, upper two-thirds of the lateral tibial surface and anterior interosseous membrane.

INNERVATION: Dorsal medial side of the first (medial) cuneiform and base of first metatarsal bone.

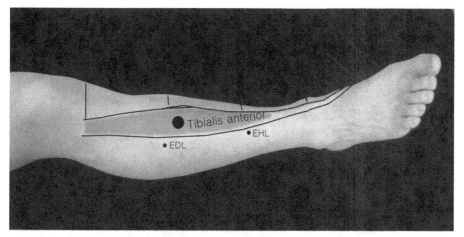

Figure 16-1. *Tibialis anterior.*

Extensor Digitorum Longus

PATIENT POSITION: Supine or side lying.

NEEDLE INSERTION: At the middle third of the leg, a needle is inserted midway between the anterior border of the tibia and the lateral border of the fibula.

ACTIVATION: Extend the toes and dorsiflex the ankle.

CLINICAL NOTES: If a needle is inserted too medially, it will be in the tibialis anterior; too deeply, it will be in the extensor hallucis longus.

INNERVATION: L5 and S1–deep peroneal nerve.

ORIGIN: Anterolateral tibial condyle, anterior proximal three-fourths of the fibula, and the adjacent anterior interosseous membrane.

INSERTION: Middle and distal phalanges of the lateral four digits, forming a membranous expansion over the dorsum of each respective metatarsal phalangeal joint where it fuses with the capsule. Near the proximal interphalangeal joint, the expansion divides into three slips. The central part of the aponeurosis continues distally to the dorsal base of the middle phalanx. Collateral slips continue to the base of the distal phalanx.

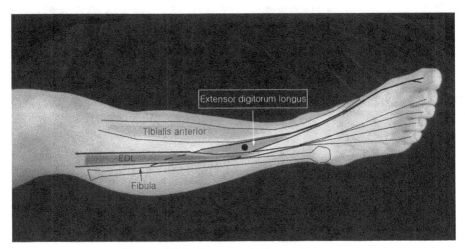

Figure 16-2. *Extensor digitorum longus.*

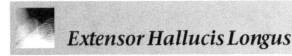

Extensor Hallucis Longus

PATIENT POSITION: Supine or side lying.

NEEDLE INSERTION: At the junction between the middle and lower third of the tibia and at the space between the tendons of tibialis anterior and extensor digitorum longus. The extensor digitorum longus tendon may be pushed laterally and the needle advanced toward the anterior surface of the fibula, with extension of the big toe and ankle dorsiflexion.

CLINICAL NOTES: This muscle is commonly tested to assess L5 radiculopathy and foot drop. The muscle lies deep partly to the tibialis anterior and extensor digitorum longus.

INNERVATION: L5, S1–peroneal part of sciatic nerve–common peroneal nerve–deep peroneal nerve.

ORIGIN: Middle third of anterior surface of fibula and the adjacent anterior interosseous membrane.

INSERTION: Dorsum of the base of the distal phalanx of the big toe.

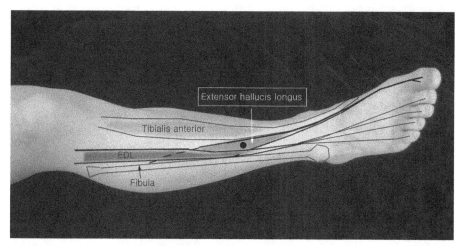

Figure 16-3. *Extensor hallucis longus.*

Peroneus Longus

PATIENT POSITION: Side lying or supine.

NEEDLE INSERTION: At 5 to 10 centimeters inferior from the fibula neck, place two fingers (thumb and index) over the anterior and lateral surfaces of the fibula, insert the needle into the space between the two fingers, and advance it toward the fibula.

ACTIVATION: Plantar flexion of the ankle and eversion of the foot.

CLINICAL NOTES: In common peroneal neuropathy at the fibular head, this muscle is often less involved than the tibialis anterior. If inserted too medially, the needle will be in the extensor digitorum longus; too posteriorly, it will be in the soleus or gastrocnemius. This muscle covers the lateral surface of the fibula.

INNERVATION: L5 and S1–peroneal portion of sciatic nerve–common peroneal nerve–superficial peroneal nerve.

ORIGIN: Head and proximal two-thirds of the lateral surface of the fibula.

INSERTION: Lateral aspect of the base of the first metatarsal bones and medial (first) cuneiform.

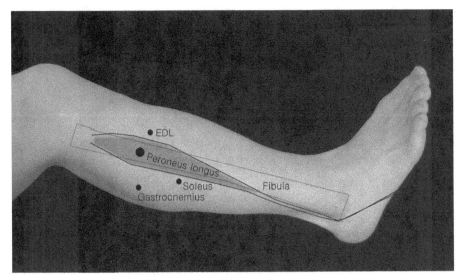

Figure 16-4. *Peroneus longus.*

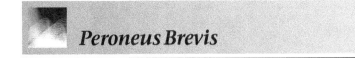
Peroneus Brevis

PATIENT POSITION: Supine or side lying.

NEEDLE INSERTION: At the anterolateral border of the fibula, the needle is inserted at the junction of the middle and lower thirds of the fibula. The proximal part of this muscle lies deep to the peroneus longus.

ACTIVATION: Plantar flexion of the ankle and eversion of the foot.

INNERVATION: L5 and S1–superficial peroneal nerve.

ORIGIN: Distal two-thirds of the lateral surface of the fibula and intermuscular fascia.

INSERTION: Dorsal lateral aspect of the base of the fifth metatarsal bone.

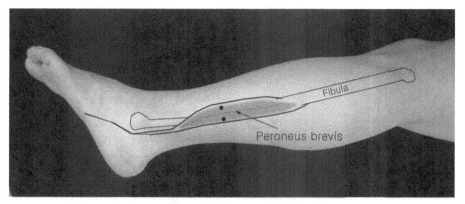

Figure 16-5. *Peroneus brevis.*

Gastrocnemius

PATIENT POSITION: Supine or side lying, or prone.

NEEDLE INSERTION: This muscle has two heads: the medial and lateral. The medial and lateral heads are divided approximately by a line drawn between the midway of popliteal crease and the Achilles tendon at the ankle. Both heads are superficial and easily recognized. The needle is inserted at the center of the muscle belly in the head of each side.

ACTIVATION: Plantar flexion of the ankle with the knee extended.

CLINICAL NOTES: The gastrocnemius is the most superficial muscle of the calf.

This muscle covers most of the soleus muscle. The medial head is easily tested even in the supine position, and it is more frequently examined than the lateral head. If the needle is inserted too deeply, it could be any muscle depending on the direction and depth: soleus, flexor digitorum longus, flexor hallucis longus, or tibialis posterior.

INNERVATION: S1, S2–sciatic nerve (tibial portion)–tibial nerve.

ORIGIN:

1. Lateral head: proximal aspect of the lateral femoral condyle.
2. Medial head: popliteal surface of the femur proximal to the medial epicondyle.

INSERTION: Achilles tendon to the calcaneus (common tendon with soleus).

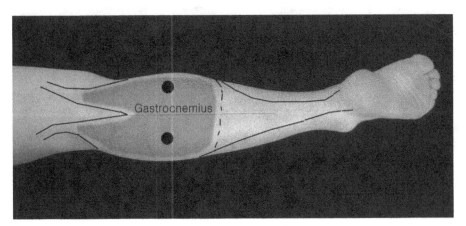

Figure 16-6. *Gastrocnemius.*

Soleus

PATIENT POSITION: Side lying or prone.

NEEDLE INSERTION: From the medial side of the calf in a side-lying position, insert the needle just below and at the anterior aspect of the lower margin of the gastrocnemius muscle belly.

ACTIVATION: Plantar flexion of the ankle.

CLINICAL NOTES: Broad, flat muscle located deep to the gastrocnemius.

MEDIAL APPROACH: If the needle is inserted too medially or too deeply, it could be in either flexor digitorum longus or tibialis posterior.

LATERAL APPROACH: If inserted too deeply, the needle will be in the flexor hallucis longus.

INNERVATION: S1, S2–sciatic nerve–tibial nerve.

ORIGIN:

1. Fibular head: proximal posterior upper third of the fibula.
2. Tibial head: proximal third of the posterior tibia.

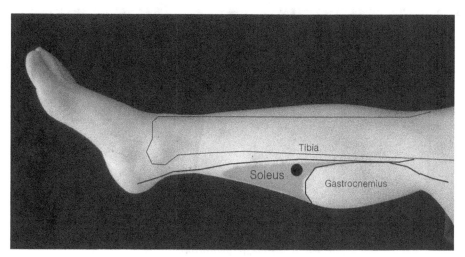

Figure 16-7. *Soleus.*

INSERTION: Achilles tendon to the calcaneus (common tendon with gastrocnemius).

 Flexor Digitorum Longus

PATIENT POSITION: Supine.

NEEDLE INSERTION: At the midway point of the calf, insert the needle just posterior and off the medial border of the tibia. Advance it toward the posterior surface of the tibia.

ACTIVATION: Flex the lateral four toes with plantar flexion and inversion of the foot.

INNERVATION: L5, S1–sciatic nerve–tibial nerve.

ORIGIN: Middle third of posterior surface of the tibia.

INSERTION: Four tendons to the plantar surfaces of the base of the terminal phalanx of digits two through five.

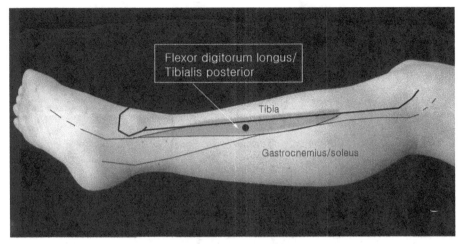

Figure 16-8. *Flexor digitorum longus.*

 Tibialis Posterior

PATIENT POSITION: Supine.

NEEDLE INSERTION: Insert the needle at the midpoint between the tibia and fibula at the middle third of the leg anteriorly and advance it through either the tibialis anterior or the extensor digitorum longus posteriorly toward the interosseous membrane connecting the tibia and fibula. After passing the interosseous membrane, the needle may reach the tibialis posterior. It requires a long needle, about the same length as the distance between the anterior and medial borders of tibia. The authors believe this approach is more accurate and perhaps safer, as it may avoid penetrating the large neurovascular structures that are located posteriorly to the tibialis posterior.

ACTIVATION: Plantar flexion of the ankle and inversion of the foot.

CLINICAL NOTES[1]: The tibialis posterior is the deepest muscle of the posterior compartment group of calf muscle. Posteriorly, there are neurovascular structures, soleus, and gastrocnemius; medially, flexor digitorum longus; laterally, flexor hallucis longus; anteriorly, interosseous membrane, part of tibialis anterior, extensor digitorum longus, tibia, and fibula. It is one of the important muscles to assess L5 radiculopathy. With one needle stick, you may check two different muscles (tibialis anterior and posterior), which are innervated by the

---

[1] Lee HJ, Bach JR, DeLisa JA: Standardization in nerve conduction study. *Am J Phys Med Rehabil* 1990;69:126–127.

same L5 root but are innervated by two different peripheral nerves (deep peroneal nerve and tibial nerve).

INNERVATION: L5 and S1–tibial nerve.

ORIGIN: Lateral aspect of the posterior tibia, proximal two-thirds of the medial posterior fibula, posterior surface of the interosseous membrane, and the intermuscular septum.

INSERTION: Navicular tuberosity, sustentaculum tali, and the three cuneiforms, cuboid, and plantar surface of bases of second, third, and fourth metatarsals.

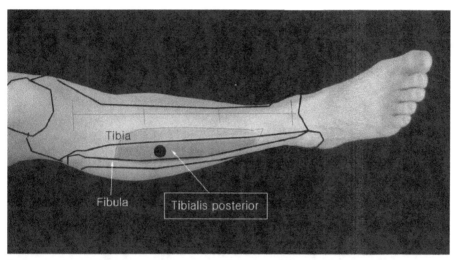

A

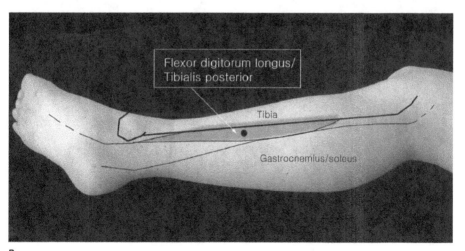

B

Figure 16-9. *Tibialis posterior.*

Flexor Hallucis Longus

PATIENT POSITION: Side lying on the opposite side or prone.

NEEDLE INSERTION: Insert the needle close to the posterior surface of the fibula at the midhalf of the calf laterally.

ACTIVATION: Flex the big toe with the plantar flexion of the ankle.

INNERVATION: S2, S3–tibial nerve.

ORIGIN: Distal two-thirds of the posterior surface of the fibula and adjacent interosseous membrane.

INSERTION: Plantar surface of the base of the distal phalanx of the big toe.

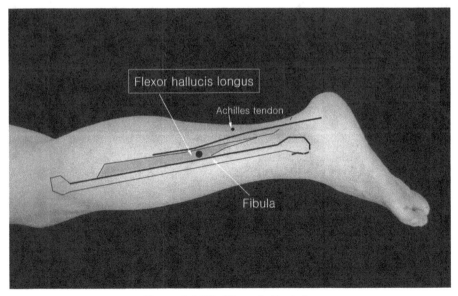

Figure 16-10. *Flexor hallucis longus.*

CHAPTER 17

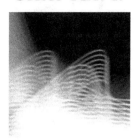

The Anterior Thigh

Iliopsoas

PATIENT POSITION: Supine with the hip slightly flexed and the knee in a comfortable position.

NEEDLE INSERTION: Note the femoral artery, anterior superior iliac spine (ASIS), and inguinal ligament. Insert the needle midway between the femoral artery (recognized by palpation of pulse) and ASIS, but just below the inguinal ligament.

ACTIVATION: Flex, adduct, and externally rotate the thigh.

CLINICAL NOTES: The lumbar plexus is located within this muscle and the femoral artery descends through the psoas major and then runs between it and the iliacus. If the needle is inserted too laterally, it will reach the sartorius.

INNERVATION: The iliacus is the most proximal muscle innervated by the femoral nerve (L2, L3), whereas the psoas major is innervated by ventral rami of the first, second, and third lumbar spinal nerves.

ORIGIN: Psoas major from bodies and transverse processes of the 12th thoracic and all the lumbar vertebrae; iliacus from the superior aspect of the iliac fossa.

INSERTION: Lesser trochanter of the femur.

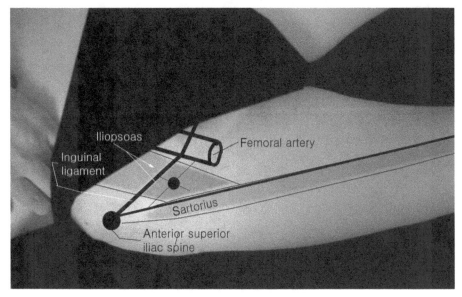

Figure 17-1. *Iliopsoas.*

Pectineus

PATIENT POSITION: Supine.

NEEDLE INSERTION: Palpate the femoral artery pulse in the inguinal area and insert the needle about 1 centimeter (cm) medial to the artery and below the inguinal fossa. If inserted too deeply, the needle will be in the obturator externus: too medially, in the gracilis or adductor longus.

ACTIVATION: Ask the patient to flex and adduct the hip.

CLINICAL NOTES: Flat, quadrilateral-shaped muscle occasionally innervated by the obturator or accessory obturator nerve.

INNERVATION: L2, L3–femoral nerve.

ORIGIN: Pectineal line of the pubis.

INSERTION: From lesser trochanter to the linea aspera of the femur.

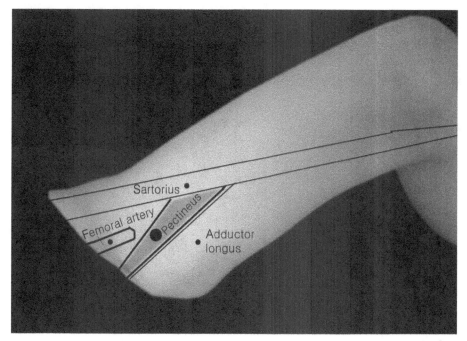

Figure 17-2. *Pectineus.*

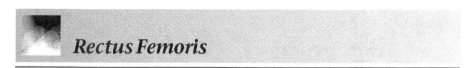

Rectus Femoris

PATIENT POSITION: Supine with the knee extended.

NEEDLE INSERTION: Insert the needle at the middle third of the femur anteriorly and halfway between the medial and lateral border of the thigh.

ACTIVATION: Flex the hip with the knee extended.

CLINICAL NOTES: Flat, spindle-shaped muscle. It is the only "quadriceps" muscle that crosses two joints. If the needle is inserted too deeply, it will be in the vastus intermedius.

INNERVATION: L2, L3, L4–femoral nerve.

ORIGIN: Anterior inferior iliac spine, upper lip of acetabulum, and fibrous capsule of the hip joint.

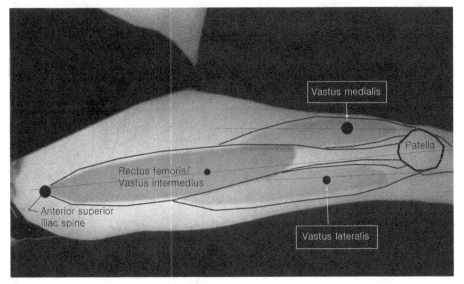

Figure 17-3. *Rectus femoris.*

INSERTION: Base of the patella and by the patella ligament into the tibial tuberosity.

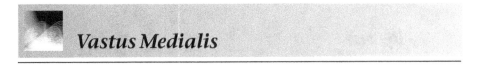

Vastus Medialis

PATIENT POSITION: Supine with the knee extended.

NEEDLE INSERTION: Insert the needle at 5 to 10 cm straight above the medial border of the patella.

ACTIVATION: Extend the knee. Ask the patient to push the kneecap down on the examination table.

CLINICAL NOTES: Located on the medial aspect of the anterior thigh. This muscle is often used for femoral nerve conduction.

INNERVATION: L2, L3, L4–femoral nerve.

ORIGIN: Medial lip of the linea aspera of the femur; intertrochanteric line of the femur and medial intermuscular septum.

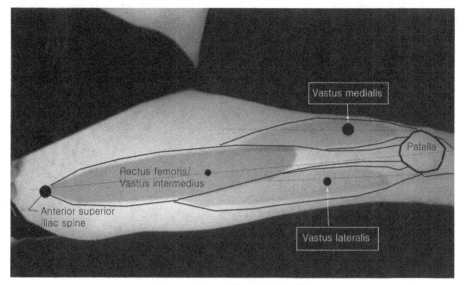

Figure 17-4. *Vastus medialis.*

INSERTION: Medial aspect of the patella and by the patellar ligament into the tibial tuberosity. Some horizontal fibers insert into the lower part of the medial border of the patella.

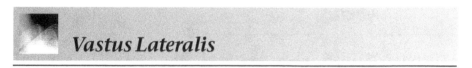

Vastus Lateralis

PATIENT POSITION: Supine.

NEEDLE INSERTION: Insert the needle at the junction of the middle and lower third of the thigh straight above the lateral border of the patella.

ACTIVATION: Extend the knee.

CLINICAL NOTES: It is a broad, thick muscle and is the largest part of the quadriceps group. It is located on the lateral aspect of the anterior thigh.

INNERVATION: L2, L3, L4–femoral nerve.

ORIGIN: Linea aspera of the femur, greater trochanter of the femur, and intertrochanteric line of the femur.

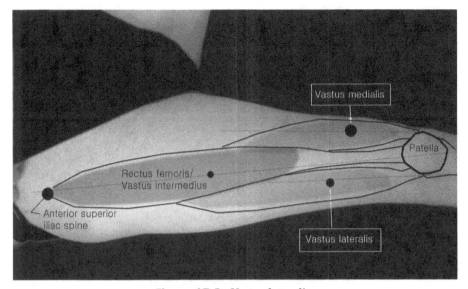

Figure 17-5. *Vastus lateralis.*

INSERTION: Lateral aspect of the patella and by the patellar ligament into the tibial tuberosity.

Sartorius

PATIENT POSITION: Supine with the hip flexed, abducted and externally rotated, and the knee flexed. Place the testing leg over the opposite leg.

NEEDLE INSERTION: Note the ASIS and medial condyle of the femur. Insert the needle 5 to 10 cm distal to ASIS in a line drawn between the ASIS and the medial condyle.

ACTIVATION: Flex, externally rotate and abduct the hip, and flex the knee.

CLINICAL NOTES: It is the longest muscle in the body and it has the longest fibers. It descends obliquely across the front and medial sides of the thigh. If the needle is inserted too medially, it will be in the iliopsoas: too deeply, rectus femoris: too laterally, in the tensor fascia lata.

INNERVATION: L2, L3, L4–femoral nerve.

ORIGIN: Anterior superior iliac spine.

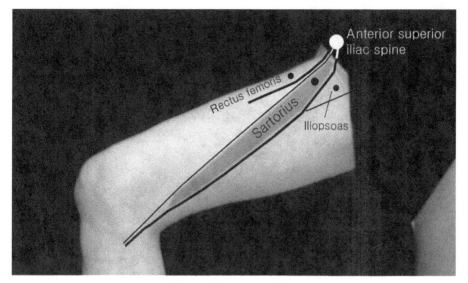

Figure 17-6. *Sartorius.*

INSERTION: Upper medial surface of the tibia, anterior to the insertion of the gracilis and the semitendinosus.

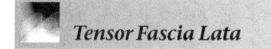

Tensor Fascia Lata

PATIENT POSITION: Side lying or supine.

NEEDLE INSERTION: Insert the needle 3 to 4 cm posterior along the line of the iliac crest from the ASIS and 5 to 10 cm inferior directly from the iliac crest toward the front of the greater trochanter of the femur.

ACTIVATION: Abduct and internally rotate the hip or abduct the hip with the knee extended.

CLINICAL NOTES: It is a thin muscle at its origin that becomes thicker at its insertion into the iliotibial tract. It is triangular and is enclosed between the two layers of the fascia lata.

INNERVATION: L4, L5, S1–superior gluteal nerve.

ORIGIN: Lateral surface of iliac crest posterior to the anterior superior iliac spine.

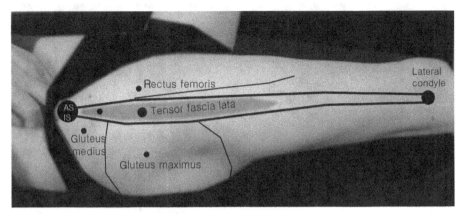

Figure 17-7. *Tensor fascia lata.*

INSERTION: Iliotibial tract to the lateral condyle of the tibia.

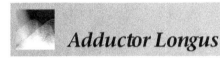

Adductor Longus

PATIENT POSITION: Supine with the hip abducted, slightly flexed, and the knee flexed. The testing leg is placed over the opposite leg.

NEEDLE INSERTION: Insert the needle at the junction of the upper and middle third of the medial thigh in a space between the sartorius and gracilis muscle.

ACTIVATION: Adduct the thigh from the patient position described above.

INNERVATION: L2, L3, L4–obturator nerve.

ORIGIN: Pubic tubercle.

INSERTION: Medial lip of the lower two-thirds of the linea aspera of the femur.

Gracilis

PATIENT POSITION: Supine with the hip flexed, abducted, and externally rotated.
　　The testing leg is placed over the opposite leg.

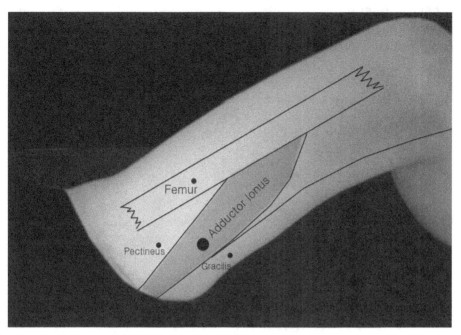

Figure 17-8. *Adductor longus.*

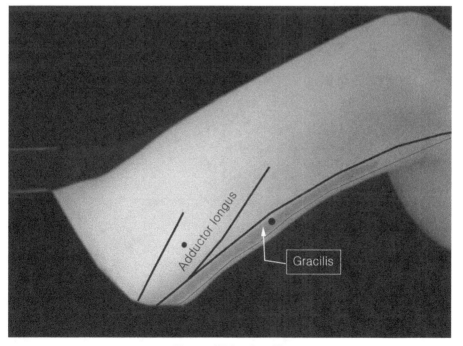

Figure 17-9. *Gracilis.*

NEEDLE INSERTION: In the patient position described above, insert the needle at the proximal one-third of the most medial side of the thigh where a cord-like, tight muscle belly is palpable.

ACTIVATION: Raise the thigh against resistance from the patient position described above (flexion and adduction of the hip).

CLINICAL NOTES: It is a superficial, thin, flat, strap-like muscle on the medial side of the knee and thigh.

INNERVATION: L2, L3–obturator nerve.

ORIGIN: Inferior ramus of the pubis and ramus of the ischium.

INSERTION: Medial proximal end of tibia just distal to medial condyle.

 Abbreviations

ASIS, anterior superior iliac spine; cm, centimeters.

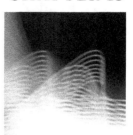

CHAPTER 18

The Buttock and Posterior Thigh

 ## Gluteus Maximus

PATIENT POSITION: Side lying or prone.

NEEDLE INSERTION: From the upper end of the intergluteal cleft, insert the needle 2 to 3 centimeters (cm) down and the same distance laterally but above the gluteal fold. The needle can also be inserted approximately 5 cm straight above the ischial tuberosity.

ACTIVATION: Extend the hip with the knee flexed. Ask the patient to squeeze his/her buttocks together.

CLINICAL NOTES: It is the largest and heaviest muscle in the body and is quadrilateral in shape. It is the most superficial muscle of the buttock region.

INNERVATION: L5, S1, S2–inferior gluteal nerve.

ORIGIN: Posterior iliac crest, posterior superior iliac spine, posterior surface of the sacrotuberous ligament, dorsum of the sacrum and coccyx, and posterior portion of the sacroiliac ligament.

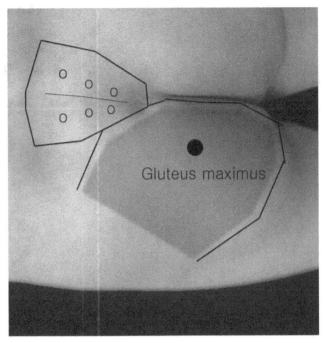

Figure 18-1. *Gluteus maximus.*

INSERTION: Gluteal tuberosity of the femur (one-fourth to one-half of total fibers).

Iliotibial band (tract) to the lateral condyle of the tibia (one-half to three-fourths of total fibers).

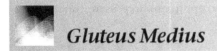 *Gluteus Medius*

PATIENT POSITION: Side lying or prone.

NEEDLE INSERTION: Note a line drawn between the iliac crest and greater trochanter of the femur. Insert the needle about 5 cm inferior from the iliac crest. If inserted too inferiorly and deeply, it will be in the gluteus minimus.

ACTIVATION: Abduct and internally rotate the thigh.

CLINICAL NOTES: Broad, thick muscle on the outer surface of the pelvis. Its posterior portion lies deep to the gluteus maximus.

INNERVATION: L5, S1–superior gluteal nerve.

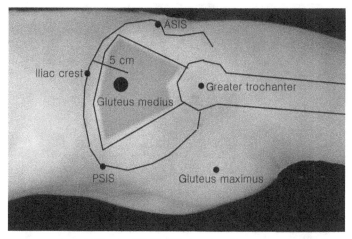

Figure 18-2. *Gluteus medius.*

ORIGIN: Outer surface of ilium between iliac crest and posterior gluteal line.

INSERTION: Greater trochanter of the femur.

 Gluteus Minimus

PATIENT POSITION: Prone or lateral recumbent.

NEEDLE INSERTION: Insert the needle at about the midposition of a line drawn between the greater trochanter of the femur and the iliac crest. This muscle is deep to the gluteus medius. Withdraw the needle a few millimeters to check the muscle when it touched the iliac bone.

ACTIVATION: Abduct the hip.

INNERVATION: L5, S1–superior gluteal nerve.

CLINICAL NOTES: Fan-shaped muscle that lies deep to the gluteus medius and is the smallest of the abductor group.

ORIGIN: Outer and lateral surface of ilium between anterior and inferior gluteal lines and margin of the greater sciatic notch.

INSERTION: Greater trochanter of the femur.

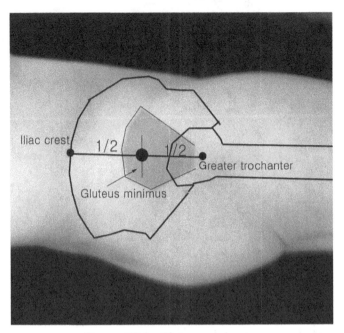

Figure 18-3. *Gluteus minimus.*

 Biceps Femoris: Long Head

PATIENT POSITION: Prone or side lying.

NEEDLE INSERTION: Insert the needle at the midpoint of a line drawn between the ischial tuberosity and tendon of the lateral hamstring at the popliteal fossa.

ACTIVATION: Extend the thigh with the leg flexed.

CLINICAL NOTES: If needle is inserted too deeply close to the femur, it will be in the short head of the biceps femoris; too medially, it will be in the medial hamstring (semimembranosus or semitendinosus).

INNERVATION: L5, S1, S2–Sciatic nerve (tibial portion).

ORIGIN: Ischial tuberosity (common tendon with the semitendinosus).

INSERTION: Head of the fibula.

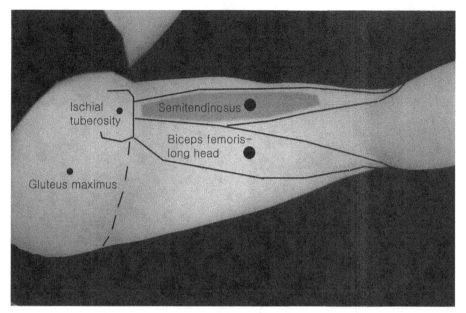

Figure 18-4. *Biceps femoris: long head.*

Biceps Femoris: Short Head

PATIENT POSITION: Prone or side lying.

NEEDLE INSERTION: Insert the needle immediately lateral or medial to the tendon of the biceps femoris, long head at the level of the popliteal fossa or above, and advance it toward the posterior aspect of the femur. Or, insert the needle parallel to the posterior surface of the distal femur between the iliotibial band and the biceps long head tendon.

ACTIVATION: Flex the knee.

CLINICAL NOTES: The short head may be congenitally absent. Foot drop may be complicated by a lesion of a peripheral nerve, frequently the common peroneal nerve at the head of the fibula or peroneal portion of the sciatic nerve in the thigh. In a patient with foot drop, this muscle should be examined to localize the nerve lesion at the fibula head or in the thigh.

INNERVATION: L5, S1–common peroneal portion of the sciatic nerve.

ORIGIN: Linear aspera of the femur.

INSERTION: Head of the fibula.

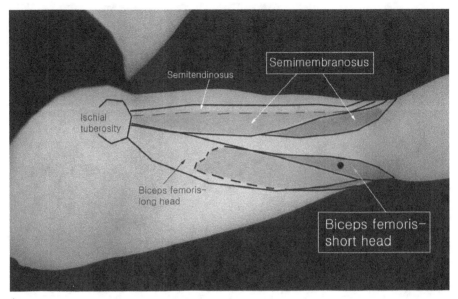

A

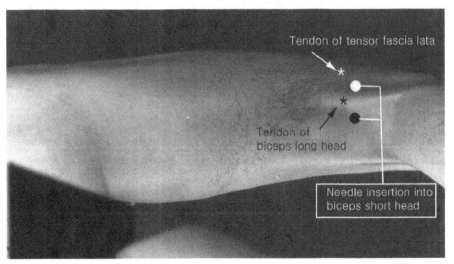

B

Figure 18-5. *Biceps femoris: short head.*

 Semitendinosus

PATIENT POSITION: Prone or side lying.

NEEDLE INSERTION: Insert the needle midway between the ischial tuberosity and the medial hamstring tendons at the popliteal fossa.

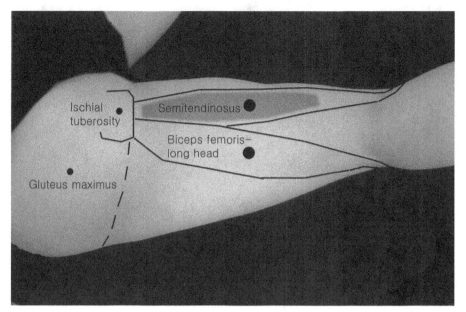

Figure 18-6. *Semitendinosus.*

ACTIVATION: Extend the thigh with the knee flexed.

CLINICAL NOTES: This muscle is fusiform in shape and is the most superficial of the hamstring group. If the needle is inserted too laterally, it will be in the biceps femoris: too deeply, it will be in the semimembranosus.

ACTIVATION: Flex the knee and extend the hip.

INNERVATION: L5, S1–tibial portion of the sciatic nerve.

ORIGIN: Ischial tuberosity, from a common tendon with the long head of the biceps femoris.

I: Medial surface of the upper tibia, posterior to the insertion of the sartorius and gracilis.

Semimembranosus

PATIENT POSITION: Prone or side lying.

NEEDLE INSERTION: The needle is inserted immediately lateral to the tendon of the semitendinosus at the level of the popliteal fossa or above.

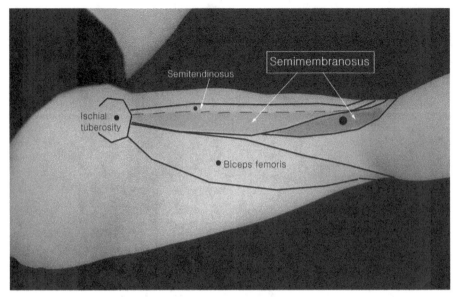

Figure 18-7. *Semimembranosus.*

CLINICAL NOTES: The proximal half of this muscle is deep to the semitendinosus and the long head of the biceps femoris.

ACTIVATION: Flex and internally rotate the flexed knee and extend the hip.

INNERVATION: L5, S1, S2–tibial portion of the sciatic nerve.

ORIGIN: Ischial tuberosity.

INSERTION: Posteromedial aspect of the medial tibial condyle. A heavy band comes off the site of the insertion and runs obliquely upward and laterally, blending with the posterior capsule of the knee joint to form the oblique popliteal ligament.

 Abbreviation

cm, centimeters.

CHAPTER 19

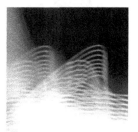

The Trunk

 ## *Diaphragm*

PATIENT POSITION: Supine.

NEEDLE INSERTION[1]

Bolton's methods: One of several interspaces between the medial clavicular and anterior axillary lines in the lower costal margins. A monopolar needle is inserted just above the costal margin at a right angle to the chest wall. As the needle advances, recordings can be made through the muscles of the chest wall (e.g., external oblique or rectus abdominus, external and internal costal muscles) and then finally, the diaphragm.

Saadeh et al.:[2] The needle is inserted at the point where the paramidclavicular line (the line drawn halfway between the jugular notch of the sternum and the lateral border of the clavicle) intersects the lower costal margin at the ninth rib cartilage. The needle slowly advances through the skin and abdominal muscle, closely hugging the posterior aspect of the chest wall, while the examiner's free hand depresses the abdominal wall. A 50-millimeter-long monopolar needle is recommended.

[1] Bolton CF: AAEM Minimonography no. 40: Clinical Neurophysiology of the respiratory system. *Muscle & Nerve* 1993;16:809–818.
[2] Saadeh PB, Crisafulli CF, Bosner J, Wolf E: Needle electromyography of the diaphragm: A new technique. *Muscle & Nerve* 1993;16:15–20.

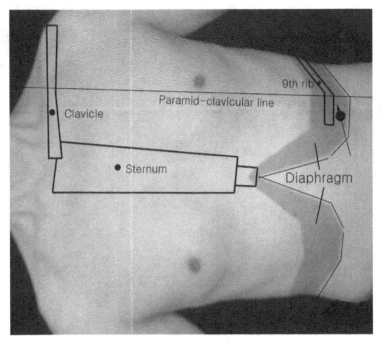

Figure 19-1. *Diaphragm.*

ACTIVATION: Regular breathing.

CLINICAL NOTES: Potential complications: pneumothorax, pneumoperitonium, bleeding. Examined for C3, C4 radiculopathy and phrenic neuropathy. Contraindication: severe obesity, marked abdominal distension.

INNERVATION: C3, C4, C5–phrenic nerve (right and left).

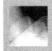 *Rectus Abdominalis*

PATIENT POSITION: Supine.

NEEDLE INSERTION: Insert the needle transversely from near the midclavicular line (or linea semilunaris) toward the linea alba in the abdominal wall.

Depending on the thickness of the subcutaneous fat, it may need a few centimeters insertion of the needle electrode to reach the muscle from the skin.

CLINICAL NOTES: Long strap-like muscles that extend the length of the front of the abdomen. These are paired muscles separated by the linea alba that

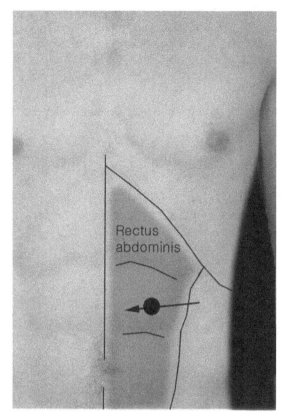

Figure 19-2. *Rectus abdominalis.*

lie under the anterior layer of the rectus sheet. Examined for lower thoracic radiculopathy and lower intercostal neuropathy, etc.

ACTIVATION: Flex the trunk.

INNERVATION: T6 (T5)–T12–Lower six thoracic nerves (intercostal).

ORIGIN: Pubic symphysis, pubic crest.

INSERTION: Fifth, sixth, and seventh costal cartilages, anterior aspect of the xyphoid process.

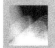 *Lumbosacral and Cervical Paraspinal Muscles/Multifidi*

PATIENT POSITION: Lateral decubitus with neck fully flexed. The neck is comfortably supported with a pillow. This position is preferable to the prone position.

NEEDLE INSERTION: Note the most prominent spinous process (C7) with the neck fully flexed. At 2 to 3 centimeters lateral to the spinous process, the needle advances directly toward the transverse process until it strikes the transverse process and is withdrawn a bit and redirected toward the groove to check the multifidus.

ACTIVATION: Ask the patient to extend his/her neck gently while checking motor unit activities.

INNERVATION: Cervical dorsal rami of the corresponding spinal nerves.

ORIGIN AND INSERTION: Transverse processes to spinous processes, the muscle fascicles are obliquely placed in relation to the vertebral column and extended two to four segments in length.

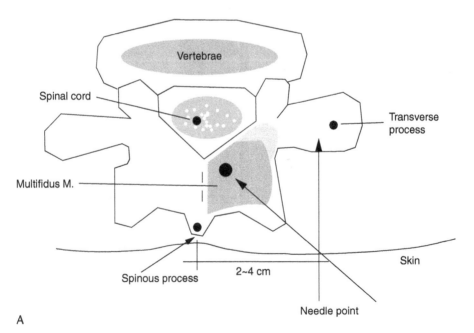

A

Figure 19-3. *Lumbosacral and cervical paraspinal muscles/multifidi.*

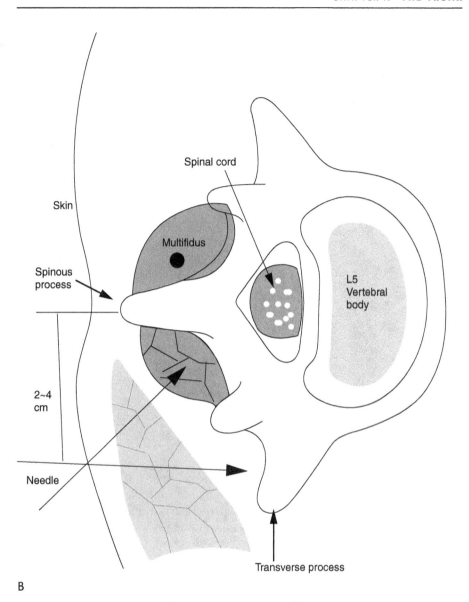

B

Figure 19-3. (*Continued*)

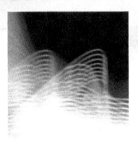

CHAPTER 20

The Pelvis

External Anal Sphincter

PATIENT POSITION: Side lying on the opposite side or supine.

NEEDLE INSERTION: Insert the gloved index finger into the rectum to guide the direction of the needle into the external anal sphincter. Insert the needle parallel to the inserted finger at the junction between the mucosal membrane and the skin of the external anal sphincter (mucocutaneous junction). It is preferable to insert the needle at a 6 o'clock or 9 o'clock direction.

ACTIVATION: Ask the patient to sqeeze the examiner's inserted gloved finger or ask the patient to act like they are defecating to obtain relaxation.

CLINICAL NOTES: This muscle is often tested in lesions of the cauda equina or conus medullaris including the pudendal nerve and S2, S3, and S4.

INNERVATION: S2, S3, S4–sacral plexus–pudendal nerve.

ORIGIN: Apex of coccyx and anococcygeal raphe.

INSERTION: Muscle fibers decussate around the anus and meet anteriorly in the central point of the perineum and the deep surface of the skin.

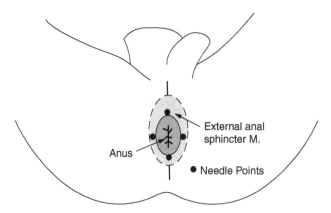

Figure 20-1. *External anal sphincter.*

Bulbocavernosus (Bulbospongiosus)

PATIENT POSITION: Supine, hip flexed and abducted (thigh spread apart), knee flexed.

NEEDLE INSERTION: It is a superficial, small, and thin layer of muscle. It is preferable to use a small needle electrode.

MALE: About midway between the root of the penis (corpus spongiosum penis) and anus, a few millimeters lateral to the median line of the perineum. Use a very short needle, and insert it at a sharp angle vertically.

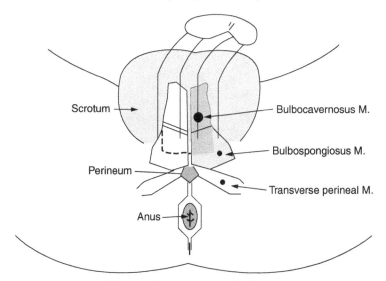

Figure 20-2. *Bulbocavernosus (Bulbospongiosus).*

ACTIVATION: Ask the patient to tighten all perineal and thigh muscles (as if to arrest defecation).

INNERVATION: S2, S3, S4–pudendal nerve.

ORIGIN: In males, median raphe and perineal body; in females, surrounds the orifice of the vagina.

INSERTION:

Male: Upper surface of the corpus spongiosum penis.

CHAPTER 21

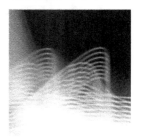

The Head and Neck

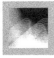 *Frontalis*

PATIENT POSITION: Supine with head slightly turned (tilted) to the opposite side.

NEEDLE INSERTION: The muscle is flat and extremely thin. Insert a short and small needle into the muscle at a 10- to 20-degree angle to the skin (relatively sharp angle) approximately at the midline between the front hair line and the eyebrow.

ACTIVATION: Ask the patient to raise the eyebrows or wrinkle the forehead.

CLINICAL NOTES: Normal motor unit action potential amplitude and duration in this muscle are usually small and short. It is often difficult to differentiate from fibrillation potentials. It also fires rapidly.

INNERVATION: Facial nerve (C VII).

ORIGIN AND INSERTION: From the scalp to above the eyebrow.

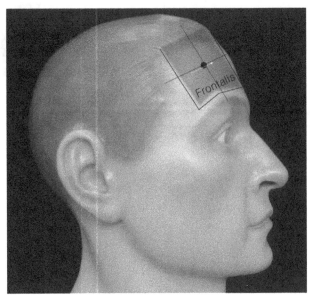

Figure 21-1. *Frontalis.*

 Orbicularis Oculi

PATIENT POSITION: Supine with head slightly tilted to the opposite side.

NEEDLE INSERTION: Before inserting the needle, make sure of the orbital fossa and its lateral, upper, and inferior borders. Insert the needle at about 1.5 centimeters (cm) from the lateral bony margin of the orbital fossa and direct it upward or downward obliquely. Insert and advance the needle at a relatively sharp angle because the muscle layer is extremely thin and superficial.

ACTIVATION: Close eyelids.

CLINICAL NOTES: Important muscle from a cosmetic (facial expression) and functional (eye closure) standpoint after facial paralysis. Black and blue markings may result from needling. A firm compression with dry cotton or gauze may be necessary after the needle is removed.

INNERVATION: Facial nerve (C VII).

ORIGIN: Nasal part of the frontal bone, frontal process of the maxilla, and anterior surface of the medial palpebral ligament.

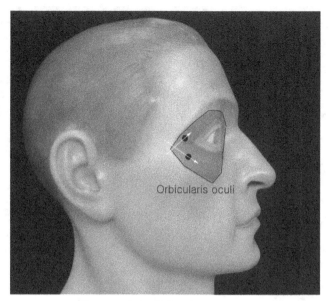

Figure 21-2. *Orbicularis oculi.*

INSERTION: Muscle fibers surround the circumference of the orbit, spread downward on the check, and blend with adjacent structures.

 Orbicularis Oris

PATIENT POSITION: Supine with the head slightly tilted to the opposite side.

NEEDLE INSERTION: Insert the needle 0.5 to 1 cm below or above the mouth angle and gradually advance it toward the midline while having the patient pucker his/her lips.

ACTIVATION: Ask the patient to whistle or pucker the lips.

CLINICAL NOTES: Rare, but isolated neuropathy of superior or inferior bucccal branches of facial nerve may be seen. Therefore, both upper and lower parts of this muscle may need to be tested separately.

INNERVATION: Facial nerve (C VII).

ORIGIN: Numerous strata of muscle fibers surrounding the orifice of the mouth, derived in part from other facial muscles.

INSERTION: External skin and mucous membrane.

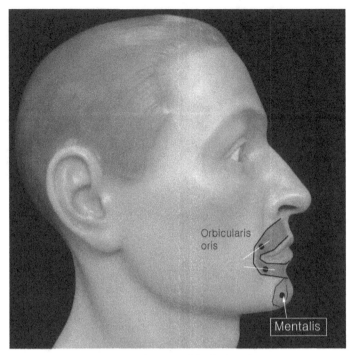

Figure 21-3. *Orbicularis oris.*

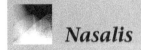 *Nasalis*

PATIENT POSITION: Supine and head tilted slightly to the opposite side.

NEEDLE INSERTION: About a half centimeter down from the ridge of nose, insert the needle parallel to the midportion of the side wall of the nostril toward the root of the nose. This muscle is extremely thin and superficial. Insert a very small needle at a sharp angle.

ACTIVATION: Widen the aperture of the nostril either by deep inspiration through the nose or by force expiration through the nostril while compressing to shut the other with a finger.

INNERVATION: Facial nerve (C VII).

ORIGIN: Maxilla.

INSERTION: Ala of nose and aponeurosis of opposite side of nasalis.

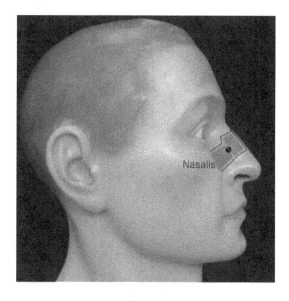

Figure 21-4. *Nasalis.*

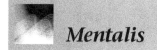 *Mentalis*

PATIENT POSITION: Supine with the chin up.

NEEDLE INSERTION: Insert the needle 0.5 to 1 cm lateral to the midline of the chin and from the lower border of the mandible. Advance it gradually upward.

ACTIVATION: Ask the patient to raise and protrude his/her lower lip

INNERVATION: Mandibular branch of the facial nerve (C VII).

ORIGIN: Incisive fossa of the mandible.

INSERTION: Skin of the chin.

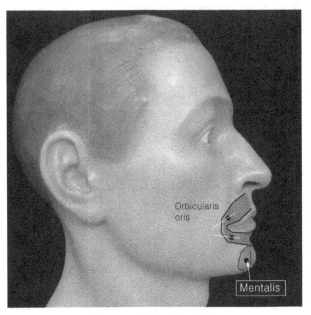

Figure 21-5. *Mentalis.*

 Auricularis Posterior

PATIENT POSITION: Supine with the head turned to the opposite side of the examination, side lying, or sitting.

NEEDLE INSERTION: This muscle is superficial and extremely thin. By pulling the ear forward, a fold is made at the midportion of the posterior aspect of the pinna. The needle is inserted into the fold (muscle under skin crease). A voluntary contraction is very difficult but you may observe the motor unit action potentials by pulling the ear lobe forward or backward.

CLINICAL NOTES: This muscle may be normal if facial neuropathy may result from a lesion distal to the styloid foramen (e.g., parotid gland abscess).

INNERVATION: Facial nerve (C VII).

ORIGIN: Mastoid portion of the temporal bone.

INSERTION: Ponticulus on the eminentia conchae.

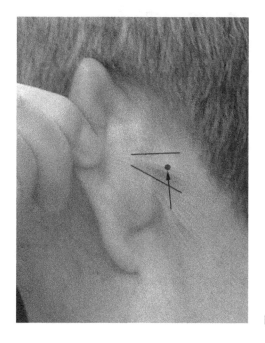

Figure 21-6. *Auricularis posterior.*

 Temporalis

PATIENT POSITION: Supine with the head turned to the opposite side.

NEEDLE INSERTION: The muscle is thin and superficial. Insert a small needle at the level of the eyebrow and advance it toward the temporal area at a relatively sharp angle to the skin (10 to 20 degrees).

ACTIVATION: Ask the subject to clench his/her teeth.

CLINICAL NOTES: Examined for trigeminal neuropathy (mandibular division).

INNERVATION: Trigeminal nerve (C V).

ORIGIN: Temporal fossa and fascia.

INSERTION: Coronoid process and anterior border of the ramus of the mandible.

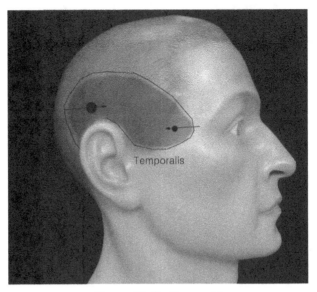

Figure 21-7. *Temporalis.*

 Masseter

PATIENT POSITION: Supine and with the head turned to the opposite side.

NEEDLE INSERTION: Note the ramus of the mandible and its jaw angle. To palpate this muscle bulk near the jaw angle, ask the subject to clench his/her mouth. Insert the needle over the muscle belly near the jaw angle or at the midpoint between the zygomatic arch and angle of the mandible.

ACTIVATION: Clench his/her teeth.

CLINICAL NOTES: Examined for trigeminal neuropathy. Avoid injuring the parotid gland that is located near the ear lobe and the mandibular angle area.

INNERVATION: Trigeminal nerve (C V).

ORIGIN: Zygomatic process of the maxilla and anterior two-thirds of zygomatic arch.

INSERTION: Lateral surface of the ramus and angle of the mandible.

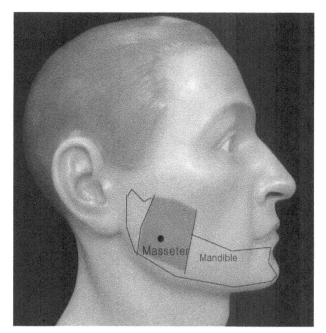

Figure 21-8. *Masseter.*

Cricothyroid

PATIENT POSITION: Supine with the head in midline and the neck in slight extension.

NEEDLE INSERTION[1]: The needle is inserted at the level of the superior border and just off the midline of the cricoid cartilage. The needle is directed superiorly and laterally toward the thyroid cartilage, while the patient is vocalizing.

CLINICAL NOTES: Make sure of the anatomic landmarks (e.g., thyroid cartilage, cricoid cartilage) before inserting the needle. The muscle is so thin that it requires a very small and short electrode to test it. Phonation is necessary to activate the motor units.

INNERVATION: Superior laryngeal nerve, branch of the vagus nerve (C X).

---

[1] Rodriquez AA, Simpson DM: 1996 AAEM Course E: Approach to the patient with bulbar symptoms—Case illustrations.

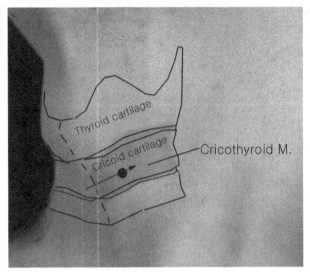

Figure 21-9. *Cricothyroid.*

ORIGIN: Front and lateral parts of the outer surface of the cricoid cartilage.

INSERTION: Posterior part of the lower border of the thyroid cartilage.

 Sternocleidomastoid

PATIENT POSITION: Supine.

NEEDLE INSERTION: Palpate the midportion of the muscle belly, while rotating the head to the opposite side, or while flexing the head to the same shoulder. Hold the medial and lateral borders of the muscle belly by the thumb and index fingers at the midportion and insert the needle.

ACTIVATION: Tilt the head toward the shoulder of the same side, or rotate the head toward the opposite side.

CLINICAL NOTES[1]: Examined for accessory neuropathy, often occurring after radical neck dissection. Advance the needle with care because there are many neurovascular structures under this muscle.

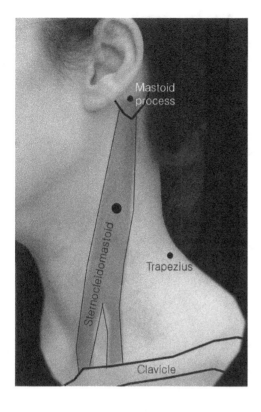

Figure 21-10. *Sternocleidomastoid.*

INNERVATION

Accessory nerve (C XI).

C2, C3, C4 (ventral rami).

ORIGIN: Sternum and medial one-third of clavicle.

INSERTION: Lateral surface of the mastoid process and lateral half of the superior nuchal line of the occipital bone.

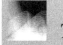 *Tongue*

PATIENT POSITION: Supine with the head in midline and the neck in slight extension.

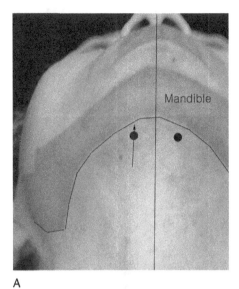

Figure 21-11. *Tongue.*

NEEDLE INSERTION

1. The examiner's gloved fingers hold the patient's tongue after asking the patient to stick out his/her tongue. The needle is inserted on the side of the tongue.

2. Head is in extension. A needle is inserted 2 to 3 cm lateral to the tip of the chin and just off the inner side of the mandibular bone. The needle should pass through the mylohyoid and geniohyoid muscles to reach the tongue and genioglossus.

ACTIVATION: Ask the patient to stick his/her tongue out (protrudes its apex from the mouth).

INNERVATION: Hypoglossal nerve (C XII).

ORIGIN

Genioglossus muscle: Upper genial tubercle on the inner surface of the symphysis of the mandible.

INSERTION: Hyoid bone.

 Abbreviation

cm, centimeters.

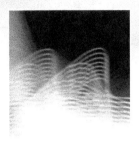

CHAPTER 22

Anatomy

Segmental Innervation of Muscles

Upper Extremity		
Muscle	*Peripheral nerve*	*Spinal segment*
Sternocleidomastoid	Spinal accessory	C2, 3
Trapezius	Spinal accessory	C3, 4
Diaphragm	Phrenic	C3, 4, 5
Levator scapulae (LS)	Nerve to LS	C3, 4
Rhomboid	Dorsal scapular	C4, 5
Supraspinatus	Suprascapular	C5, 6
Infraspinatus	Suprascapular	C5, 6
Teres major	Subscapular	C6, 7
Teres minor	Axillary	C5, 6
Serratus anterior	Long thoracic	C5, 6, 7
Latissimus dorsi	Thoracodorsal	C6, 7, 8
Pectoralis major	Lateral and Medial pectoral	C5, 6, 7, 8, and T1
Deltoid	Axillary	C5, 6
Biceps	Musculocutaneous	C5, 6
Coracobrachialis	Musculocutaneous	C5, 6
Brachialis	Musculocutaneous	C5, 6
Triceps	Radial	C6, 7, 8
Anconeous	Radial	C7, 8

Upper Extremity (*continued*)

Muscle	Peripheral nerve	Spinal segment
Brachioradialis	Radial	C5, 6
Extensor carpi radialis	Radial	C6, 7
Extensor digitorum	Radial	C7, 8
Extensor carpi ulnaris	Radial	C7, 8
Extensor pollicis longus	Radial	C7, 8
Abductor pollicis longus	Radial	C7, 8
Extensor indicis	Radial	C7, 8
Supinator	Radial	C5, 6
Pronator teres	Median	C6, 7
Flexor carpi radialis	Median	C6, 7
Palmaris longus	Median	C7, 8
Flexor digitorum sublimis	Median	C7, 8, and T1
Flexor digitorum	Median	C8 and T1
profundus	Ulnar	C8 and T1
Pronator quandratus	Median	C8 and T1
Flexor pollicis longus	Median	C8 and T1
Flexor carpi ulnaris	Ulnar	C7, 8
Abductor digiti minimi	Ulnar	C8 and T1
Adductor pollicis	Ulnar	C8 and T1
Interossei	Ulnar	C8 and T1
Lumbricals:		
1st and 2nd	Median	C8 and T1
3rd and 4th	Ulnar	C8 and T1
Abductor pollicis brevis	Median	C8 and T1
Opponens pollicis	Median (Ulnar)	C8 and T1

Lower Extremity

Muscle	Peripheral nerve	Spinal segment
Iliopsoas	Femoral	L2, 3
Sartorius	Femoral	L2, 3
Quadriceps	Femoral	L2, 3, 4
Adductor longus	Obturator	L2, 3, 4
Adductor magnus	Obturator and Sciatic	L2, 3, 4
Gracilis	Obturator	L2, 3
Tensor fascia lata	Superior gluteal	L4, 5, and S1
Gluteus medius	Superior gluteal	L4, 5, and S1
Gluteus maximus	Inferior gluteal	L5, S1, and 2
Biceps femoris:		
Short head	Sciatic (common peroneal)	L5, S1 and 2
Long head	Sciatic (tibial)	L5, S1 and 2
Semitendinosus	Sciatic (tibial)	L5, S1 and 2
Semimembranosus	Sciatic (tibial)	L5, S1 and 2

Lower Extremity (*continued*)

Muscle	*Peripheral nerve*	*Spinal segment*
Tibialis anterior	Deep peroneal	L4, 5
Extensor digitorum longus	Deep peroneal	L5 and S1
Extensor hallucis longus	Deep peroneal	L5 and S1
Extensor digitorum brevis	Deep peroneal	L5, S1 and 2
Peroneus longus	Superficial peroneal	L5 and S1
Gastrocnemius	Tibial	S1, 2
Soleus	Tibial	S1, 2
Flexor digitorum longus	Tibial	L5, S1 and 2
Flexor hallucis longus	Tibial	S2, 3
Tibialis posterior	Tibial	L5 and S1
Abductor hallucis	Medial plantar	S2, 3
Flexor digitorum brevis	Medial plantar	S2, 3
Abductor digiti minimi	Lateral plantar	S2, 3
Lumbricals	Medial and Lateral plantar	S2, 3

Myotome

C5
  Deltoid
  Supraspinatus
  Infraspinatus
  Teres major
  Biceps brachii
  Brachioradialis
  Rhomboid
C6
  Brachioradialis
  Biceps
  Pronator teres
  Flexor carpi radialis
  Extensor carpi radialis
  Supinator
  Serratus anterior
C7
  Triceps
  Anconeous
  Extensor carpi radialis longus

  Extensor digitorum
  Pronator teres
  Flexor carpi radialis
  Flexor digitorum superficialis
  Serratus anterior
C8 and T1
  Extensor carpi ulnaris
  Extensor indicis
  Flexor carpi ulnaris
  Flexor digitorum profundus
  Abductor pollicis brevis
  Pronator quadratus
  Flexor pollicis longus
  Flexor pollicis brevis
  Abductor digiti minimi
  First dorsal interosseous
L23
  Ilicus
  Vastus medialis
  Vastus lateralis

Myotome (*continued*)

Rectus femoris	Flexor digitorum longus
Adductor longus	Extensor hallucis longus
L4	Extensor digitorum brevis
Vastus medialis	Medial hamstring
Vastus lateralis	Gluteus medius
Rectus femoris	Tensor fascia lata
Tibialis anterior	S1
Medial hamstring	Gastrocnemius
Gluteus medius	Soleus
Tensor fascia lata	Tibialis posterior
L5	Abductor hallucis
Tibialis anterior	Peroneous longus
Tibialis posterior	Extensor digitorum brevis
Peroneus longus	Lateral hamstring
Extensor digitorum longus	Gluteus maximus

Root Search for Cervical Radiculopathy

Muscle	Root	Nerve
Deltoid	C5, 6	Axillary
Biceps	C5, 6	Musculocutaneous
Pronator teres	C6, 7	Median
Triceps	C6, 7, 8	Radial
First dorsi interosseous	C8, T1	Ulnar
Cervical paraspinals	Posterior ramus	

Root Search for Lumbosacral Radiculopathy

Muscle	Root	Nerve
Vastus lateralis	L2, 3, 4	Femoral
Tibialis anterior	L4, 5	Deep peroneal
Peroneous longus	L5, S1	Superficial peroneal
Gastrocnemius (medial)	S1, 2	Tibial
Gluteus maximus	S1, 2	Inferior gluteal
Lumbosacral paraspinals	Posterior ramus	

Glossary of Terms

A wave A *compound muscle action potential* that follows the *M wave*, evoked consistently from a muscle by submaximal electric stimuli and frequently abolished by *supramaximal stimuli*. Its *amplitude* is similar to that of an *F wave*, but the *latency* is more constant. Usually occurs before the F wave, but may occur afterward. Thought to be due to extra *discharges* in the nerve, *ephapses*, or axonal branching. This term is preferred over *axon reflex, axon wave,* or *axon response.* Compare with the *F wave.*

absolute refractory period See *refractory period.*

accommodation In neuronal physiology, a rise in the *threshold* transmembrane *depolarization* required to initiate a *spike,* when depolarization is slow or a subthreshold depolarization is maintained. In the older literature, the observation that the final intensity of current applied in a slowly rising fashion to stimulate a nerve was greater than the intensity of a pulse of current required to stimulate the same nerve. The latter may be largely an *artifact* of the nerve sheath and bears little relation to true accommodation as measured intracellularly.

accommodation curve See *strength-duration curve.*

acoustic myography The recording and analysis of sounds produced by contracting muscle. The muscle *contraction* may be produced by stimulation of the nerve supply to the muscle or by volitional *activation* of the muscle.

action potential (AP) The brief regenerative electric *potential* that propagates along a single axon or muscle fiber membrane. An all-or-none phenomenon; whenever the *stimulus* is at or above *threshold,* the action potential generated has a constant size and configuration. See also *compound action potential, motor unit action potential.*

activation 1) In physiology, a general term for the initiation of a process. 2) The process of *motor unit action potential* firing. The force of muscle *contraction* is determined by the number of *motor units* and their *firing rate.*

activation procedure A technique used to detect defects of neuromuscular transmission during *repetitive nerve stimulation* testing. Most commonly a sustained voluntary *contraction* is performed to elicit *facilitation* or *postactivation depression.* See also *tetanic contraction.*

active electrode Synonymous with *exploring electrode.* See *recording electrode.*

acute inflammatory neuropathy An acute, monophasic *polyneuropathy.* Characterized by a time course of progression to maximum deficit within 4 weeks of onset of symptoms. Most common clinical presentation is an ascending sensory-motor *neuropathy.* Electrodiagnostic studies most commonly reveal evidence for *demyelination,* but *axonal degeneration* also occurs. Distinguish from *chronic inflammatory demyelinating polyradiculoneuropathy (CIDP).* See also *Guillain-Barré syndrome.*

adaptation A decline in the *frequency* of the *spike discharge* as typically recorded from sensory axons in response to a maintained *stimulus.*

ADEMG Abbreviation for *automatic decomposition electromyography.*

AEP Abbreviation for *auditory evoked potential.*

afterdischarge 1) The continuation of *action potentials* in a neuron, axon, or muscle fiber following the termination of an applied *stimulus.* 2) The continuation of firing of *muscle action potentials* after cessation of voluntary *activation*—for example, in *myotonia.*

afterpotential The membrane *potential* between the end of the *spike* and the time when the membrane potential is restored to its resting value. The membrane during this period may be depolarized or hyperpolarized at different times.

akinesia Lack or marked *delay* of intended movement, often observed in patients with Parkinson's disease. Often used synonymously with *bradykinesia.*

amplitude With reference to an *action potential,* the maximum *voltage* difference between two points, usually *baseline*-to-peak or peak-to-peak. By convention, the amplitudes of *potentials* that have an initial negative deflection from the baseline, such as the *compound muscle action potential* and the *antidromic sensory nerve action potential*, are measured from baseline to the most negative peak. In contrast, the amplitudes of a *compound sensory nerve action potential, motor unit potential, fibrillation potential, positive sharp wave, fasciculation potential*, and most other action potentials are measured from the most positive peak to the most negative peak.

amplitude decay The percent change in the *amplitude* of the *M wave* or the *compound sensory nerve action potential* between two different stimulation points along the nerve. Decay = 100 × (amplitude$_{distal}$ − amplitude$_{proximal}$) / amplitude$_{distal}$. Useful in the evaluation of *conduction block*. Abnormal decay without increased *temporal dispersion* may indicate a conduction block.

anodal block A local block of nerve conduction caused by membrane *hyperpolarization* under a stimulating *anode*. Does not occur in routine clinical studies, since it is possible for the anode to routinely result in nerve *depolarization* if sufficient current intensities are used.

anode The positive terminal of an electric current source. See *stimulating electrode*.

antidromic Propagation of a nerve impulse in the direction opposite to physiologic conduction; e.g., conduction along *motor nerve* fibers away from the muscle and conduction along sensory fibers away from the spinal cord. Contrast with *orthodromic*.

AP Abbreviation for *action potential*.

artifact (also artefact) A *voltage* change generated by a biologic or nonbiologic source other than the ones of interest. The *stimulus artifact* (or *shock artifact*) represents cutaneous spread of stimulating current to the *recording electrode* and the *delay* in return to *baseline*, which is dependent on the ability of filters to respond to high voltage. Stimulus artifacts may precede or overlap the activity of interest. *Movement artifact* refers to a change in the recorded activity caused by movement of the recording electrodes.

asterixis A quick involuntary movement caused by a brief lapse in tonic muscle *activation*. It can be appreciated only during voluntary movement. Is usually irregular but can be rhythmic and confused with action *tremor*.

ataxia Clumsiness of movement. Specific features include dysmetria (incorrect distance moved) and dysdiadochokinesis (irregularity of attempted rhythmic movements). Most commonly due to a disorder of the cerebellum or proprioceptive sensory system. Referred to, respectively, as cerebellar ataxia and sensory ataxia.

auditory evoked potential (AEP) Electric *waveforms* of biologic origin elicited in response to sound stimuli. Classified by their *latency* as short-latency *brainstem auditory evoked potential (BAEP)* with a latency of up to 10 ms, middle-latency with a latency of 10 to 50 ms, and long-latency with a latency of over 50 ms. See *brainstem auditory evoked potential*.

automatic decomposition EMG (ADEMG) computerized method for extracting individual *motor unit action potentials* from an *interference pattern*.

averager See signal *averager*.

averaging A method for extracting time-locked *potentials* from random background *noise* by sequentially adding traces and dividing by the total number of traces.

axon reflex Use of term discouraged as it is incorrect. No *reflex* is thought to be involved. See preferred term, *A wave*.

axon response See preferred term, *A wave*.

axon wave See *A wave*.

axonal degeneration Degeneration of the segment of a nerve distal to the cell body with preferential distal pathology.

axonotmesis Nerve injury characterized by axon and myelin sheath disruption with supporting connective tissue preservation, resulting in *axonal degeneration* distal to the injury site. Compare *neurapraxia, neurotmesis*.

backaveraging *Averaging* a signal that occurs in a time epoch preceding a triggering event. Often used to extract a time-locked EEG signal preceding voluntary or involuntary movement, usually triggered by the onset of the *EMG* activity of the movement. An example is the *Bereitschaftspotential*.

backfiring *Discharge* of an *antidromically* activated motor neuron.

BAEP Abbreviation for *brainstem auditory evoked potential*.

BAER Abbreviation for *brainstem auditory evoked response*. See preferred term, *brainstem auditory evoked potential*.

baseline 1) The *potential* recorded from a biologic system while the system is at rest.

2) A flat trace on the recording instrument; an equivalent term, *isoelectric line*, may be used.

benign fasciculation potential A *firing pattern* of *fasciculation potentials* occurring in association with a clinical syndrome of *fasciculations* in an individual with a non-progressive neuromuscular disorder. Use of term discouraged.

BER Abbreviation for *brainstem auditory evoked responses*. See preferred term, *brainstem auditory evoked potentials*.

Bereitschaftspotential (BP) A component of the *movement-related cortical potential*. The slowly rising negativity in the EEG preceding voluntary movement. The German term means "readiness potential." Has two *phases* called BPI and BP2 or BP and NS (negative slope). See *backaveraging*.

biphasic action potential An *action potential* with one *baseline* crossing, producing two *phases*.

biphasic end-plate activity See *end-plate activity (biphasic)*.

bipolar needle electrode *Recording electrode* that measures *voltage* between two insulated wires cemented side-by-side in a steel cannula. The bare tips of the electrodes are flush with the level of the cannula, which may serve as a ground.

bipolar stimulating electrode See *stimulating electrode*.

bizarre high-frequency discharge See preferred term, *complex repetitive discharge*.

bizarre repetitive discharge See preferred term, *complex repetitive discharge*.

bizarre repetitive potential See preferred term, *complex repetitive discharge*.

blink reflex See *blink responses*.

blink responses *Compound muscle action potentials* evoked from orbicularis oculi muscles as a result of brief electric or mechanical *stimuli* applied to the cutaneous area innervated by the supraorbital (or less commonly, the infraorbital) branch of the trigeminal nerve. Typically, there is an early compound muscle action potential (*R1 wave*) ipsilateral to the stimulation site with a *latency* of about 10 ms and a bilateral late compound muscle action potential (*R2 wave*) with a latency of approximately 30 ms. Generally, only the R2 wave is associated with a visible *contraction* of the muscle. The configuration, *amplitude, duration*, and latency of the two components, along with

the sites of recording and stimulation, should be specified. The R1 and R2 waves are oligosynaptic and polysynaptic brainstem *reflexes*, respectively. Together they are called the *blink reflex*. The afferent arc is provided by the sensory branches of the trigeminal nerve and the efferent arc is provided by facial nerve motor fibers.

blocking Term used in *single fiber electromyography* to describe dropout of one or more components of the *potential* during sequential firings. If more than one component drops out simultaneously it is described as concomitant blocking. Usually seen when *jitter* values exceed 80 to 100 μs. A sign of abnormal neuromuscular transmission, which may be due to primary *neuromuscular transmission disorders*, such as *myasthenia gravis* and other myasthenic syndromes. Also seen as a result of degeneration and reinnervation in *neuropathies* or *myopathies*. Concomitant blocking may be generated by a split muscle fiber or failure of conduction at an axon branch serving several muscle fibers.

BP Abbreviation for *Bereitschaftspotential*.

brachial plexus An anatomical structure that is formed by the spinal roots from C5 to T1, traverses the shoulder region, and culminates in the named peripheral nerves in the arm. It is composed of roots, trunks, divisions, cords, and terminal nerves.

bradykinesia Slowness of movement, often observed in patients with Parkinson's disease. Often used synonymously with *akinesia*.

brainstem auditory evoked potential (BAEP) Electric *waveforms* of biologic origin elicited in response to sound stimuli. Normally consists of a sequence of up to seven waves, designated I to VII, which occur during the first 10 ms after the onset of the *stimulus* and have positive polarity at the vertex of the head.

brainstem auditory evoked response (BAER, BER) See preferred term, *brainstem auditory evoked potentials*.

BSAP Abbreviation for brief, small, abundant potentials. (See *BSAPP*). Use of term is discouraged.

BSAPP Abbreviation for brief, small, abundant, polyphasic *potentials*. Used to describe a *recruitment pattern* of brief *duration*, small *amplitude*, overly abundant, polyphasic *motor unit action potentials*, with respect to the amount of force generated; usually a minimal *contraction*. Use of term discouraged. Quantitative measurements of motor unit action potential duration, amplitude, numbers of *phases,* and *recruitment frequency* are preferred. See *motor unit action potential.*

carpal tunnel syndrome A *mononeuropathy* affecting the median nerve at the wrist. As the nerve passes through the carpal tunnel, a space bounded dorsally by the bones of the wrist, laterally by the forearm flexor tendons, and volarly by the transverse carpal ligament, it is subject to compression by any of these structures. Repetitive hand and wrist movement is thought to contribute to the compression.

C reflex An abnormal *reflex response* representing the electrophysiologic correlate of sensory evoked *myoclonus.* The term "C" was chosen to indicate that the reflex might be mediated in the cerebral cortex. This is sometimes, but not always, true.

c/s (also cps) Abbreviation for *cycles per second.* See preferred term, *Hertz (H₂).*

cathode The negative terminal of an electric current source. See *stimulating electrode.*

center frequency The mean or median *frequency* of a *waveform* decomposed by *frequency analysis.* Employed in the study of muscle *fatigue.*

central electromyography Use of electrodiagnostic recording techniques to study *reflexes* and the control of movement by the spinal cord and brain. See *electrodiagnosis.*

central motor conduction The time taken for conduction of *action potentials* in the central nervous system from motor cortex to alpha motoneurons in the spinal cord or brainstem. Calculated from the *latencies* of the *motor evoked potentials* produced by *transcranial magnetic stimulation* or *transcranial electrical stimulation,* subtracting the time for peripheral conduction.

chorea Clinical term used to describe irregular, random, brief, abrupt, involuntary movements of the head or limbs due to a disorder of the basal ganglia. Most commonly observed in patients with Huntington's disease and Sydenham's chorea.

chronaxie (also chronaxy) See *strength-duration curve.*

chronic inflammatory demyelinating polyradiculoneuropathy (CIDP) A *polyneuropathy* or *polyradiculoneuropathy* characterized by generalized *demyelination*

of the peripheral nervous system. In most cases there is also a component of *axonal degeneration.* Some cases are associated with a monoclonal gammopathy of undetermined significance (MGUS). Distinguish from *acute inflammatory neuropathy.*

clinical electromyography Term used commonly to describe the scientific methods of recording and analysis of biologic electrical *potentials* from human peripheral nerve and muscle. See preferred term, *electrodiagnostic medicine.*

CMAP Abbreviation for *compound muscle action potential.*

coaxial needle electrode See synonym, *concentric needle electrode.*

collision When used with reference to *nerve conduction studies,* the interaction of two *action potentials* propagated toward each other from opposite directions on the same nerve fiber so that the *refractory periods* of the two potentials prevent propagation pass each other.

complex motor unit action potential A *motor unit action potential* that is polyphasic or serrated. See preferred terms, *polyphasic action potential* or *serrated action potential.*

complex repetitive discharge A type of *spontaneous* activity. Consists of a regularly repeating series of complex polyphasic or serrated *potentials* that begin abruptly after *needle electrode* movement or spontaneously. The potentials have a uniform shape, *amplitude,* and *discharge frequency* ranging from 5 to 100 *Hz.* The discharge typically terminates abruptly. May be seen in both myopathic and neurogenic disorders, usually chronic. Thought to be due to ephaptic excitation of adjacent muscle fibers in a cyclic fashion. This term is preferred to *bizarre high frequency discharge, bizarre repetitive discharge, bizarre repetitive potential, pseudomyotonic discharge,* and *synchronized fibrillation.* See also *ephapse and ephaptic transmission.*

compound action potential A *potential* or *waveform* resulting from the summation of multiple individual axon or *muscle fiber action potentials.* See *compound mixed nerve action potential, compound motor nerve action potential, compound nerve action potential, compound sensory nerve action potential,* and *compound muscle action potential.*

compound mixed nerve action potential A *compound nerve action potential* recorded from a *mixed nerve* when an electric *stimulus* is applied to a segment of the nerve that contains both afferent and efferent fibers. The *amplitude, latency, duration,* and *phases* should be noted.

compound motor nerve action potential (compound motor NAP) A *compound nerve action potential* recorded from efferent fibers of a *motor nerve* or a motor branch of a *mixed nerve.* Elicited by stimulation of a motor nerve, a motor branch of a mixed nerve, or a ventral nerve root. The *amplitude, latency, duration,* and number of *phases* should be noted. Distinguish from *compound muscle action potential.*

compound muscle action potential (CMAP) The summation of nearly synchronous *muscle fiber action potentials* recorded from a muscle, commonly produced by stimulation of the nerve supplying the muscle either directly or indirectly. *Baseline*-to-peak *amplitude, duration, and latency* of the negative *phase* should be noted, along with details of the method of stimulation and recording. Use of specific named *potentials* is recommended, e.g., *M wave, F wave, H wave, T wave, A wave,* and *R1 or R2 wave (blink responses).*

compound nerve action potential (compound NAP) The summation of nearly synchronous *nerve fiber action potentials* recorded from a nerve trunk, commonly produced by stimulation of the nerve directly or indirectly. Details of the method of stimulation and recording should be specified, together with the fiber type *(sensory, motor,* or *mixed nerve).*

compound sensory nerve action potential (compound SNAP) A *compound nerve action potential* recorded from the afferent fibers of a *sensory nerve,* a sensory branch of a *mixed nerve,* or in response to stimulation of a sensory nerve or a dorsal nerve root. May also be elicited when an adequate *stimulus* is applied synchronously to sensory receptors. The *amplitude, latency, duration,* and configuration should be noted. Generally, the amplitude is measured as the maximum peak-to-peak *voltage* when there is an initial positive deflection or from *baseline*-to-peak when there is an initial negative deflection. The latency is measured as either the time to the initial deflection or the negative peak, and the duration as the interval from the first deflection of the *waveform* from the baseline to its final return to the baseline. Also referred to by the less preferred terms *sensory response, sensory potential,* and *SNAP.*

concentric needle electrode *Recording electrode* that measures an electric *potential* difference between a centrally insulated wire and the cannula of the needle through which it runs.

conditioning stimulus See *paired stimuli.*

conduction block Failure of an *action potential* to propagate past a particular point in the nervous system, whereas conduction is possible below the point of the block. Documented by demonstration of a reduction in the area of a *compound muscle action potential* greater than that normally seen with stimulation at two different points on a nerve trunk; anatomic variations of nerve pathways and technical factors related to nerve stimulation must be excluded as the cause of the reduction in area.

conduction distance The length of nerve or muscle over which conduction is determined, customarily measured in centimeters or millimeters.

conduction time See *conduction velocity.*

conduction velocity (CV) Speed of propagation of an *action potential* along a nerve or muscle fiber. The nerve fibers studied (motor, sensory, autonomic, or *mixed nerve)* should be specified. For a nerve trunk, the maximum conduction velocity is calculated from the *latency* of the *evoked potential* (muscle or nerve) at maximal or supramaximal intensity of stimulation at two different points. The distance between the two points *(conduction distance)* is divided by the difference between the corresponding latencies *(conduction time).* The calculated result is the conduction velocity of the fastest fibers and is usually expressed as meters per second (m/s). As commonly used, refers to the *maximum conduction velocity.* By specialized techniques, the conduction velocity of other fibers can also be determined and should be specified, e.g., *minimum conduction velocity.*

congenital myasthenia A heterogeneous group of genetic disorders of the neuromuscular junction manifest by muscle weakness and *fatigue.*

contraction A voluntary or involuntary reversible muscle shortening that may or may not be accompanied by *action potentials* from muscle. Contrast the term *contracture.*

contraction fasciculation Clinical term for visible twitching of a muscle with weak voluntary or postural *contraction,* which has the appearance of a *fasciculation.* More likely to occur in neuromuscular disorders in which the *motor unit* territory is enlarged and the tissue covering the muscle is thin, but may also be observed in normal individuals.

contracture 1) Fixed resistance to stretch of a shortened muscle due to fibrous connective tissue changes and loss of sarcomeres in the muscle. Limited movement of a joint may be due to muscle contracture or to fibrous connective tissue changes in the joint. Contrast with *contraction,* which is a rapidly reversible painless shortening of the muscle. 2) The prolonged, painful, electrically silent, and involuntary state of temporary muscle shortening seen in some *myopathies* (e.g. muscle phosphorylase deficiency).

coupled discharge See preferred term, *satellite potential.*

cps (also c/s) Abbreviation for *cycles per second.* See preferred term, *Hertz (Hz).*

cramp discharge Involuntary repetitive firing of *motor unit action potentials* at a high *frequency* (up to 150 *Hz*) in a large area of a muscle usually associated with painful muscle *contraction.* Both *discharge frequency* and number of motor unit action potentials activated increase gradually during development, and both subside gradually with cessation. See *muscle cramp.*

crossed leg palsy Synonym for *peroneal neuropathy at the knee.*

cross talk 1) A general term for abnormal communication between excitable membranes. See *ephapse* and *ephaptic transmission.* 2) Term used in *kinesiologic EMG* for signals picked up from adjacent muscles.

cubital tunnel syndrome A *mononeuropathy* involving the ulnar nerve in the region of the elbow. An *entrapment neuropathy* caused by compression of the nerve as it passes through the aponeurosis (the cubital tunnel) of the two heads of the flexor carpiulnaris approximately 1.5 to 3.5 cm distal to the medial epicondyle of the elbow. The mechanism of entrapment is presumably narrowing of the cubital tunnel during elbow flexion. See also *tardy ulnar palsy* and *ulnar neuropathy at the elbow.*

cutaneous reflex A *reflex* produced by cutaneous stimulation. There are several *phases*

to cutaneous reflexes, and, if the muscle has a background *contraction,* the phases can be seen to be inhibitory as well as excitatory.

CV Abbreviation for *conduction velocity.*

cycles per second (c/s, cps) Unit of *frequency.* See preferred term *hertz (Hz).*

decomposition EMG Synonym for *automatic decomposition EMG.*

decremental response See preferred term, *decrementing response.*

decrementing response A reproducible decline in the *amplitude* and/or area of the *M wave* of successive *responses* to *repetitive nerve stimulation.* The rate of stimulation and the total number of stimuli should be specified. Decrementing responses with disorders of neuromuscular transmission are most reliably seen with slow rates (2 to 5 *Hz*) of nerve stimulation. A decrementing response with *repetitive nerve stimulation* commonly occurs in disorders of neuromuscular transmission but can also be seen in some *neuropathies, myopathies,* and *motor neuron disease.* An *artifact* resembling a decrementing response can result from movement of the *stimulating* or *recording electrodes* during *repetitive nerve stimulation* (see *pseudodecrement*). Contrast with *incrementing response.*

delay 1) The time between the beginning of the horizontal sweep of the oscilloscope and the onset of an applied *stimulus.* 2) A synonym for an information storage device *(delay line)* used to display events occurring before a trigger signal.

delay line An information storage device used to display events that occur before a trigger signal. A method for displaying a *waveform* at the same point on a sweep from a free-running *electromyogram.*

demyelination Disease process affecting the myelin sheath of central or peripheral nerve fibers, manifested by *conduction velocity* slowing, *conduction block,* or both.

denervation potential Sometimes used as a synonym for *fibrillation potential.* Use of this term is discouraged, since fibrillation potentials can occur in the absence of denervation. See preferred term, *fibrillation potential.*

depolarization A change in the existing membrane *potential* to a less negative value. Depolarizing an excitable cell from its resting level to *threshold* typically generates an *action potential.*

depolarization block Failure of an excitable cell to respond to a *stimulus* due to preexisting *depolarization* of the cell membrane.

depth electrodes *Electrodes* that are inserted into the substance of the brain for electrophysiological recording. Most often inserted using stereotactic techniques.

dermatomal somatosensory evoked potential (DSEP) Scalp recorded *waveforms* generated from repeated stimulation of a specific dermatome. Different from typical *somatosensory evoked potentials,* which are recorded in response to stimulation of a named peripheral nerve.

discharge The firing of one or more excitable elements (neurons, axons, or muscle fibers); as conventionally used, refers to all-or-none *potentials* only. Synonymous with *action potential.*

discharge frequency The rate at which a *potential* discharges repetitively. When potentials occur in groups, the rate of recurrence of the group and rate of repetition of the individual components in the groups should be specified. See also *firing rate.*

discrete activity See *interference pattern.*

distal latency The interval between the delivery of a *stimulus* to the most distal point of stimulation on a nerve and the onset of a *response.* A measure of the conduction properties of the distal most portion of motor or sensory nerves. See *motor latency* and *sensory latency.*

double discharge Two sequential firings of a *motor unit action potential* of the same form and nearly the same *amplitude,* occurring consistently in the same relationship to one another at intervals of 2 to 20 ms. See also *multiple discharge, triple discharge.*

doublet Synonym for the preferred term, *double discharge.*

DSEP Abbreviation for *dermatomal somatosensory evoked potential.*

duration The time during which something exists or acts. 1) The interval from the beginning of the first deflection from the *baseline* to its final return to the baseline of an *action potential* or *waveform,* unless otherwise specified. If only part of the waveform is measured, the points of the measurement should be specified. For example, the duration of the *M wave* may be measured as the negative *phase* duration and refers to the interval from the deflection of the first negative phase from the baseline

to its return to the baseline. 2) The interval of the applied current or *voltage* of a single electric *stimulus.* 3) The interval from the beginning to the end of a series of recurring stimuli or action potentials.

dynamic EMG See *kinesiologic EMG.*

dyskinesia An abnormal involuntary movement of a *choreic* or *dystonic* type. The term is nonspecific and is often used in association with a modifier that describes its etiology, e.g. tardive dyskinesia or LDOPA dyskinesia.

dystonia A disorder characterized by involuntary movements caused by sustained muscle *contraction,* producing prolonged movements or abnormal postures.

E-1 Synonymous with *input terminal 1.* See *recording electrode.*

E-2 Synonymous with *input terminal 2.* See *recording electrode.*

E:I ratio In autonomic testing, the ratio of the longest electrocardiographic R-R interval during expiration to the shortest during inspiration. Primarily a measure of parasympathetic control of heart rate.

early recruitment A *recruitment pattern* that occurs in association with a reduction in the number of muscle fibers per *motor unit* or when the force generated by the fibers is reduced. At low levels of muscle *contraction* more *motor unit action potentials* are recorded than expected, and a *full interference pattern* may be recorded at relatively low levels of muscle contraction. Most often encountered in *myopathy.*

earth electrode Synonymous with *ground electrode.*

EDX Abbreviation for *electrodiagnosis.* Can also be used for electrodiagnostic and *electrodiagnostic medicine.*

electric inactivity See preferred term, *electric silence.*

electric silence The absence of measurable electric activity due to biologic or nonbiologic sources. The sensitivity and signal-to-*noise* level of the recording system should be specified.

electrocorticography Electrophysiologic recording directly from the surface of the brain. In the intraoperative setting, recordings are made of ongoing spontaneous electroencephalogram activity, or *potentials* evoked by stimulation of peripheral sensory pathways.

electrode A conducting device used to record an electric *potential (recording electrode)* or to deliver an electric current (*stimulating electrode*). In addition to the *ground electrode* used in clinical recordings, two electrodes are always required either to record an electric potential or to deliver a *stimulus*. See *ground electrode, recording electrode,* and *stimulating electrode.* Also see specific *needle electrode* configurations: *monopolar, unipolar, concentric, bifilar recording, bipolar stimulating, multilead, single fiber,* and *macro-EMG needle electrodes.*

electrodiagnosis (EDX) The scientific methods of recording and analyzing biologic electrical *potentials* from the central, peripheral, and autonomic nervous systems and muscles. See also *clinical electromyography, electromyography, electroneurography, electroneuromyography, evoked potentials, electrodiagnostic medicine, electrodiagnostic medicine consultation,* and *electrodiagnostic medicine consultant.*

electrodiagnostic medicine A specific area of medical practice in which a physician integrates information obtained from the clinical history, observations from physical examination, and scientific data acquired by recording electrical *potentials* from the nervous system and muscle to diagnose, or diagnose and treat diseases of the central, peripheral, and autonomic nervous systems, neuromuscular junctions, and muscle. See also *electrodiagnosis, electrodiagnostic medicine consultation,* and *electrodiagnostic medicine consultant.*

electrodiagnostic medicine consultant A physician specially trained to obtain a medical history, perform a physical examination, and record and analyze data acquired by recording electrical *potentials* from the nervous system and muscle to diagnose and/or treat diseases of the central, peripheral, and autonomic nervous systems, neuromuscular junction, and muscle. See also *electrodiagnosis, electrodiagnostic medicine,* and *electrodiagnostic medicine consultation.*

electrodiagnostic medicine consultation The medical evaluation in which a specially trained physician (*electrodiagnostic medicine consultant*) obtains a medical history, performs a physical examination, and integrates scientific data acquired by recording electrical *potentials* from the nervous system and muscle to diagnose and/or treat diseases of the central, peripheral, and autonomic nervous systems;

neuromuscular junction; and muscle. See also *electrodiagnosis, electrodiagnostic medicine,* and *electrodiagnostic medicine consultant.*

electromyogram The record obtained by *electromyography.*

electromyograph Equipment used to activate, record, process, and display electrical *potentials* for the purpose of evaluating the function of the central, peripheral, and autonomic nervous systems; neuromuscular junction; and muscles.

electromyographer See preferred term, *electrodiagnostic medicine consultant.*

electromyography (EMG) Strictly defined, the recording and study of *insertion, spontaneous,* and *voluntary activity* of muscle with a *recording electrode* (either a *needle electrode* for invasive *EMG* or a *surface electrode* for kinesiologic studies). The term is also commonly used to refer to an *electrodiagnostic medicine consultation,* but its use in this context is discouraged.

electroneurography (ENG) The recording and study of the *action potentials* of peripheral nerve. Synonymous with *nerve conduction studies.*

electroneuromyography (ENMG) The combined studies of *electromyography* and *electroneurography.* Synonymous with *clinical electromyography.* See preferred term *electrodiagnostic medicine consultation.*

EMG Abbreviation for *electromyography.*

end-plate activity Spontaneous electric activity recorded with a *needle electrode* close to muscle end plates. These *potentials* may have several different morphologies.

1. Monophasic: Low-*amplitude* (10 to 20 μV), short-*duration* (0.5 to 1.0 ms), negative potentials occurring in a dense, steady pattern, the exact *frequency* of which cannot be defined. These nonpropagated potentials are probably *miniature end-plate potentials* recorded extracellularly. Referred to as *endplate noise* or *sea-shell sound (sea shell roar or noise).*

2. Biphasic: Moderate-amplitude (100 to 300 μV), short-duration (2 to 4 ms), initially negative *spike* potentials occurring irregularly in short bursts with a high frequency (50 to 100 *Hz*). These propagated potentials are generated by muscle fibers excited by activity in nerve terminals. These potentials have been referred to as biphasic spike potentials, *end-plate*

spikes, and, incorrectly, *nerve potentials.* May also have a biphasic initially positive morphology.

3. Triphasic: Similar to biphasic potentials, but the *waveforms* have three *phases* with an initial positive deflection. Fire in an irregular fashion; contrast with *fibrillation potential.*

end-plate noise See *end-plate activity (monophasic).*

end-plate potential (EPP) The graded nonpropagated membrane potential induced in the postsynaptic membrane of a muscle fiber by release of acetylcholine from the presynaptic axon terminal in response to an *action potential.*

end-plate spike See *end-plate activity (biphasic).*

end-plate zone The region in a muscle where neuromuscular junctions are concentrated.

ENG Abbreviation for *electroneurography.*

ENMG Abbreviation for *electroneuromyography.*

entrapment neuropathy A *mononeuropathy* caused by compression of a nerve as it passes through an area of anatomical narrowing.

ephapse A point of abnormal communication where an *action potential* in one muscle fiber or axon can cause *depolarization* of an adjacent muscle fiber or axon to generate an action potential.

ephaptic transmission The generation of a *nerve fiber action potential* from one muscle fiber or axon to another through an *ephapse.* Postulated to be the basis for *complex repetitive discharges, myokymic discharges,* and *hemifacial spasm.*

EPSP Abbreviation for *excitatory postsynaptic potential.*

Erb's point The site at the anterolateral base of the neck where percutaneous nerve stimulation activates the axons comprising the upper trunk of the *brachial plexus.*

Erb's point stimulation Percutaneous *supraclavicular nerve stimulation* during which the upper trunk of the *brachial plexus* is activated. See the more general and preferred term, *supraclavicular nerve stimulation.*

evoked potential Electric *waveform* elicited by and temporally related to a *stimulus,* most commonly an electric stimulus delivered to a sensory receptor or nerve, or applied directly to a discrete area of the brain, spinal cord, or muscle. See *auditory evoked potential, brainstem auditory evoked potential, spinal evoked potential, somatosensory evoked potential, visual evoked potential, compound muscle action potential,* and *compound sensory nerve action potential.*

evoked potential studies Recording and analysis of electric *waveforms* of biologic origin elicited in response to electrical, magnetic, or physiological *stimuli.* Stimuli are applied to specific motor or sensory receptors, and the resulting waveforms are recorded along their anatomic pathways in the peripheral and central nervous system. A single motor or sensory modality is typically tested in a study, and the modality studied is used to define the type of study performed. See *auditory evoked potentials, brainstem auditory evoked potentials, visual evoked potentials,* and *somatosensory evoked potentials.*

evoked response Tautology. Use of term discouraged. See preferred term, *evoked potential.*

excitability Capacity to be activated by or react to a *stimulus.*

excitatory postsynaptic potential (EPSP) A local, graded *depolarization* of a neuron in response to *activation* by a nerve terminal. Contrast with *inhibitory postsynaptic potential.*

exploring electrode Synonymous with *active electrode.* See *recording electrode.*

F reflex An incorrect term for *F wave.*

F response Synonymous with *F wave.* See preferred term, *F wave.*

F wave An *action potential* evoked intermittently from a muscle by a supramaximal electric *stimulus* to the nerve due to *antidromic activation* of *motor neurons.* When compared with the maximal *amplitude* of the *M wave,* it is smaller (1% to 5% of the M wave) and has a variable configuration. Its *latency* is longer than the M wave and is variable. It can be evoked in many muscles of the upper and lower extremities, and the latency is longer with more distal sites of stimulation. Named "F" wave by Magladery and McDougal in 1950, because it was first recorded from foot muscles. Compare with the *H wave* and the *A wave.* One of the *late responses.*

facial neuropathy Clinical diagnosis of facial weakness or paralysis due to pathology affecting the seventh cranial nerve (facial nerve). Bell's palsy refers to a facial *neuropathy* due to inflammation of the facial nerve.

facilitation An increase in an electrically measured *response* following identical *stimuli*. Occurs in a variety of circumstances: 1) Improvement of neuromuscular transmission resulting in *activation* of previously inactive muscle fibers. May be identified in several ways: *Incrementing response*—a reproducible increase in the *amplitude* and area of successive *M waves* during *repetitive nerve stimulation*. *Postactivation* or *posttetanic facilitation*—Nerve stimulation studies performed within a few seconds after a brief period (2 to 60 s) of nerve stimulation producing *tetanus* or after a strong voluntary *contraction* may show changes in the configuration of the M wave(s) compared to the results of identical studies of the rested muscle as follows: a) *repair of the decrement*—a diminution of the *decrementing response* with slow rates (2 to 5 *Hz*) of repetitive nerve stimulation; b) increment after exercise—an increase in the amplitude and area of the M wave elicited by a single supramaximal stimulus. Distinguish from *pseudofacilitation*, which occurs in normal individuals in response to repetitive nerve stimulation at high rates (20 to 50 *Hz*) or after strong volitional contraction. It probably reflects a reduction in the *temporal dispersion* of the summation of a constant number of *muscle fiber action potentials* and is characterized by an increase in the amplitude of the successive M waves with a corresponding decrease in their *duration*. There is no net change in the area of the negative *phase* of successive M waves. 2) An increase in the amplitude of the *motor evoked potential* as a result of background muscle activation.

far-field A region of electrical *potential* where the isopotential *voltage* lines associated with a current source change slowly over a short distance. Some use the term far-field potential to designate a potential that does not change in *latency, amplitude*, or polarity over infinite distances; alternative designations include "boundary potential" and "junctional potential." The terms *near-field* and far-field are arbitrary designations as there are no agreed-upon criteria defining where the near-field ends and the far-field begins. Compare with *near-field*.

fasciculation The random, spontaneous twitching of a group of muscle fibers belonging to a single *motor unit*. The twitch may produce movement of the overlying skin (if in limb or trunk muscles) or mucous membrane (if in the tongue). If the motor unit is sufficiently large, an associated joint movement may be observed. The electric activity associated with the twitch is termed a *fasciculation potential*. See also *myokymia*. Historically, the term *fibrillation* was used incorrectly to describe fine twitching of muscle fibers visible through the skin or mucous membranes. This usage is no longer accepted.

fasciculation potential The electric activity associated with a *fasciculation*, which has the configuration of a *motor unit activation potential* but occurs spontaneously. Most commonly occur sporadically and are termed "single fasciculation potentials." Occasionally the potentials occur as a *grouped discharge* and are termed a brief " *repetitive discharge*." The repetitive firing of adjacent fasciculation potentials, when numerous, may produce an undulating movement of muscle (see *myokymia*). Use of the terms *benign fasciculation* and *malignant fasciculation* is discouraged. Instead, the configuration of the *potentials*, peak-to-peak *amplitude, duration*, number of *phases*, stability of configuration, and *frequency* of occurrence, should be specified.

fatigue A state of depressed responsiveness resulting from activity. Muscle fatigue is a reduction in *contraction* force following repeated voluntary contraction or electric stimulation.

fiber density 1) Anatomically, a measure of the number of muscle or nerve fibers per unit area. 2) In *single fiber electromyography*, the mean number of *muscle fiber action potentials* fulfilling *amplitude* and *rise time* criteria belonging to one *motor unit* within the recording area of a *single fiber needle electrode* encountered during a systematic search in a weakly, voluntarily contracting muscle. See also *single fiber electromyography, single fiber needle electrode*.

fibrillation The spontanus *contractions* of individual muscle fibers that are not visible through the skin. This term has been used loosely in *electromyography* for the preferred term, *fibrillation potential*.

fibrillation potential The *action potential* of a single muscle fiber occurring spontaneously or after movement of a *needle electrode*. Usually fires at a constant rate. Consists of biphasic or triphasic *spikes* of short *duration* (usually less than 5 ms) with an initial positive *phase* and a peak-to-peak *amplitude* of less than 1 mV. May also have a biphasic, initially negative phase when recorded at the site of initiation. It has an associated high-pitched regular sound described as "rain on a tin roof." In addition to this classic form, *positive sharp waves* may also be recorded from fibrillating muscle fibers when the potential arises from an area immediately adjacent to the needle electrode.

firing pattern Qualitative and quantitative descriptions of the sequence of *discharge* of electric *waveforms* recorded from muscle or nerve.

firing rate *Frequency* of repetition of a *potential*. The relationship of the frequency to the occurrence of other potentials and the force of muscle *contraction* may be described. See also *discharge frequency*.

flexor reflex A *reflex* produced by a noxious cutaneous *stimulus*, or a train of electrical stimuli, that activates the flexor muscles of a limb and thus acts to withdraw it from the stimulus. In humans, it is well-characterized only in the lower extremity.

frequency Number of complete cycles of a repetitive *waveform* in 1 second. Measured in *hertz (Hz)* or *cycles per second (cps* or *c/s)*.

frequency analysis Determination of the range of *frequencies* composing a *waveform*, with a measurement of the absolute or relative *amplitude* of each component frequency.

full interference pattern See *interference pattern*.

full wave rectified EMG The absolute value of a *raw EMG* signal. Involves inverting all the *waveforms* below the *isopotential line* and displaying them with opposite polarity above the line. A technique used to analyze *kinesiologic EMG* signals.

functional refractory period See *refractory period*.

G1, G2 Abbreviation for *grid 1* and *grid 2*.

generator In *volume conduction* theory, the source of electrical activity, such as an *action potential*. See *far-field* and *near-field*.

"giant" motor unit action potential Use of term discouraged. Refers to a *motor unit action potential* with a peak-to-peak *amplitude* and *duration* much greater than the range found in corresponding muscles in normal subjects of similar age. Quantitative measurements of amplitude and duration are preferable.

giant somatosensory evoked potential Enlarged *somatosensory evoked potentials* seen as a characteristic of cortical *reflex myoclonus* and reflecting cortical hyperexcitability.

grid 1 Synonymous with *G1, input terminal 1 (E-1)*, or *active* or *exploring electrode*. Use of the term *G1* is discouraged. See *recording electrode*.

grid 2 Synonymous with *G2, input terminal 2 (E-2)*, or *reference electrode*. Use of the term *Grid 2* is discouraged. See *recording electrode*.

ground electrode A connection from the patient to earth. Used as a common return for an electric circuit and as an arbitrary zero *potential* reference point.

grouped discharge Term used historically to describe three phenomena: (1) irregular, voluntary grouping of *motor unit action potentials* as seen in a tremulous muscular *contraction;* (2) involuntary grouping of motor unit action potentials as seen in *myokymia;* (3) general term to describe repeated firing of motor unit action potentials. See preferred term, *repetitive discharge*.

Guillain-Barré syndrome Eponym for *acute inflammatory neuropathy*. Also referred to as Landry-Guillain-Barré syndrome or Landry-Guillain-Barré-Strohl syndrome.

H reflex Abbreviation for Hoffmann reflex. See *H wave*.

H response See preferred term *H wave*.

H wave A *compound muscle action potential* with a consistent *latency* recorded from muscles after stimulation of the nerve. Regularly found in adults only in a limited group of physiologic extensors, particularly the calf muscles. Compared to the *M wave* of the same muscle, has a longer latency and thus is one of the *late responses* (see *A* and *F wave*). Most reliably elicited with a *stimulus* of long *duration* (500 to 1000 μs). A stimulus intensity sufficient to elicit a maximal amplitude M wave reduces or abolishes the H wave. Thought to be due to a spinal *reflex*, with electric stimulation of afferent fibers in the *mixed nerve* and *activation* of motor neurons to the muscle mainly through a monosynaptic connection in the spinal cord. The latency is longer with more distal sites of stimulation. The reflex and *wave* are named in honor of Hoffman's description (1918). Compare the *F wave* and *A wave*.

habituation Decrease in size of a *reflex motor response* to an afferent *stimulus* when the latter is repeated, especially at regular and recurring short intervals.

hemifacial spasm Clinical condition characterized by frequent, repetitive, unilateral, involuntary *contractions* of the facial muscles. Electrodiagnostic studies demonstrate brief *discharges* of groups of *motor unit action potentials* occurring simultaneously in several facial muscles. Occasionally high-*frequency* discharges occur.

hertz (Hz) Unit of *frequency*. Synonymous with *cycles per second*.

Hoffmann reflex See *H wave*.

hyperekplexia Clinical condition characterized by exaggerated *startle reflexes*. Startle reflexes can be exaggerated by being more extreme than expected (larger *amplitude* or more widespread) or by lack of normal *habituation* to repeated similar *stimuli*. Can be either genetic or acquired.

hyperpolarization A change in the existing membrane *potential* to a more negative value.

hypertonia See *tone*.

hypotonia See *tone*.

Hz Abbreviation for *hertz*.

impulse blocking See *blocking*.

inching A *nerve conduction study* technique consisting of applying stimuli at multiple short distance increments along the course of a nerve. This technique is used to localize an area of focal slowing or *conduction block*.

incomplete activation *Motor unit action potentials* firing, on requested maximal effort, in decreased numbers at their normal physiological rates, within the basal firing range of 5 to 10 *Hz*. Causes include *upper motor neuron syndrome*, pain on muscle *contraction*, hysteria/conversion reaction and malingering. Contrast with *reduced recruitment*.

increased insertion activity See *insertion activity*.

increment after exercise See *facilitation*.

incremental response See preferred term, *incrementing response*.

incrementing response A reproducible increase in *amplitude* and/or area of successive *M waves* to *repetitive nerve stimulation*. The rate of stimulation and the number of *stimuli* should be specified. Commonly seen in two situations. First, in normal subjects the configuration of the M wave may

change in response to repetitive nerve stimulation so that the amplitude progressively increases as the *duration* decreases, leaving the area of the M wave unchanged. This phenomenon is termed *pseudofacilitation*. Second, in *neuromuscular transmission disorders*, the configuration of the M wave may change with repetitive nerve stimulation so that the amplitude and the area of the M wave progressively increase. This phenomenon is termed *facilitation*. Contrast with *decrementing response*.

indifferent electrode Synonymous with *reference electrode*. Use of term discouraged. See *recording electrode*.

infraclavicular plexus Segments of the *brachial plexus* inferior to the divisions; includes the three cords and the terminal peripheral nerves. This clinically descriptive term is based on the fact that the clavicle overlies the divisions of the brachial plexus when the arm is in the anatomic position next to the body.

inhibitory postsynaptic potential (IPSP) A local graded *hyperpolarization* of a neuron in response to *activation* at a synapse by a nerve terminal. Contrast with *excitatory postsynaptic potential*.

injury potential 1) The *potential* difference between a normal region of the surface of a nerve or muscle and a membrane region that has been injured; also called a "demarcation," or "killed end" potential. Approximates the potential across the membrane because the injured surface has nearly the same potential as the interior of the cell. 2) In *electrodiagnostic medicine*, the term is also used to refer to the electrical activity associated with *needle electrode* insertion into muscle. See preferred terms *fibrillation potential, insertion activity*, and *positive sharp wave*.

input terminal 1 The input terminal of a differential amplifier at which negativity, relative to the other input terminal, produces an upward deflection. Synonymous with *active* or *exploring electrode, E-1* or less preferred term, *grid 1*. See *recording electrode*.

input terminal 2 The input of a differential amplifier at which negativity, relative to the other input terminal, produces a downward deflection. Synonymous with *reference electrode, E-2* or less preferred term, *grid 2*. See *recording electrode*.

insertion activity Electric activity caused by insertion or movement of a *needle* *electrode* within a muscle. The amount of the activity may be described as normal, reduced, or increased (prolonged), with a description of the *waveform* and repetition rate. See also *fibrillation potential* and *positive sharp wave*.

integrated EMG Mathematical integration of the *full wave rectified EMG* signal. Reflects the cumulative EMG activity of a muscle over time. See also *linear envelope EMG*.

interdischarge interval Time between consecutive *discharges* of the same *potential*. Measurements should be made between the corresponding points on each *waveform*.

interference Unwanted electric activity recorded from the surrounding environment.

interference pattern Electric activity recorded from a muscle with a *needle electrode* during maximal voluntary effort. A full interference pattern implies that no individual *motor unit action potentials* can be clearly identified. A reduced interference pattern (intermediate pattern) is one in which some of the individual motor unit action potentials may be identified while others cannot due to superimposition of *waveforms*. The term *discrete activity* is used to describe the electric activity recorded when each of several different motor unit action potentials can be identified in an ongoing recording due to limited superimposition of waveforms. The term *single unit pattern* is used to describe a single motor unit action potential, firing at a rapid rate (should be specified) during maximum voluntary effort. The force of *contraction* associated with the interference pattern should be specified. See also *early recruitment, recruitment pattern, reduced recruitment pattern*.

interference pattern analysis Quantitative analysis of the *interference pattern*. This can be done either in the *frequency* domain using fast Fourier transformation (FFT) or in the time domain. Can be done using a fixed load (e.g., 2 kg), at a given proportional strength (e.g., 30% of maximum) or at random strengths. The following are measured in the time domain: a) the number of *turns* per second and b) the *amplitude*, defined as the mean amplitude between peaks.

intermediate interference pattern See *interference pattern*.

international 10–20 system A system of *electrode* placement on the scalp in which electrodes are placed either 10% or 20% of the total distance on a line on the skull between the nasion and inion in the sagittal plane and between the right and left preauricular points in the coronal plane.

interpeak interval Difference between the peak *latencies* of two components of a *waveform*.

interpotential interval Time between two different *potentials*. Measurement should be made between the corresponding parts of each *waveform*.

intraoperative monitoring The use of electrophysiological stimulating and recording techniques in an operating room setting. The term is usually applied to techniques that are used to detect injury to nervous tissue during surgery or to guide the surgical procedure.

involuntary activity *Motor unit action potentials* that are not under volitional control. The condition under which they occur should be described, e.g., spontaneous or *reflex* potentials. If elicited by a *stimulus*, its nature should be described. Contrast with *spontaneous activity*.

IPSP Abbreviation for *inhibitory postsynaptic potential*.

irregular potential See preferred term, *serrated action potential*.

isoelectric line In electrophysiologic recording, the display of zero *potential* difference between the two input terminals of the recording apparatus. See *baseline*.

iterative discharge See preferred term, *repetitive discharge*.

jiggle Shape variability of *motor unit action potentials* recorded with a conventional *EMG needle electrode*. A small amount occurs normally. In conditions of disturbed neuromuscular transmission, including early reinnervation and myasthenic disorders, the variability can be sufficiently large to be easily detectable by eye. Quantitative methods for estimating this variability are not yet widely available.

jitter The variability of consecutive *discharges* of the *interpotential* interval between two *muscle fiber action potentials* belonging to the same *motor unit*. Usually expressed quantitatively as the mean value of the difference between the interpotential intervals of successive discharges (the *mean consecutive difference, MCD*). Under certain conditions, it is expressed as the mean value of the difference between interpotential intervals arranged in the order of decreasing interdischarge intervals (the *mean sorted difference, MSD*). See *single fiber electromyography*.

Jolly Test A technique named for Friedrich Jolly, who applied an electric current to excite a *motor nerve* repetitively while recording the force of muscle *contraction*. Use of the term is discouraged. Inappropriately used to describe the technique of *repetitive nerve stimulation*.

kinematics Technique for description of body movement without regard to the underlying forces. See *kinesiologic EMG*.

kinesiologic EMG The muscle electrical activity recorded during movement. Gives information about the timing of muscle activity and its relative intensity. Either *surface electrodes* or intramuscular fine *wire electrodes* are used. Synonymous with *dynamic EMG*.

kinesiology The study of movement. See *kinesiologic EMG*.

kinetics The internal and external forces affecting the moving body. See *kinesiologic EMG*.

late component (of a motor unit action potential) See preferred term, *satellite potential*.

late response A general term used to describe an *evoked potential* in motor *nerve conduction studies* having a longer *latency* than the *M wave*. Examples include *A wave, F wave*, and *H wave*.

latency Interval between a *stimulus* and a *response*. The *onset latency* is the interval between the onset of a stimulus and the onset of the *evoked potential*. The *peak latency* is the interval between the onset of a stimulus and a specified peak of the evoked potential.

latency of activation The time required for an electric *stimulus* to depolarize a nerve fiber (or bundle of fibers as in a nerve trunk) beyond *threshold* and to initiate an *action potential* in the fiber(s). This time is usually of the order of 0.1 ms or less. An equivalent term, now rarely used, is the "utilization time."

latent period See preferred term, *latency*.

linear envelope EMG Moving average of the *full wave rectified EMG*. Obtained by low pass filtering the full wave rectified EMG. See also *integrated EMG*.

linked potential See preferred term, *satellite potential*.

lipoatrophy Pathologic loss of subcutaneous fat and connective tissues overlying muscle that mimics the clinical appearance of atrophy of the underlying muscle.

long-latency reflex A *reflex* with many synapses (polysynaptic) or a long pathway (long-loop) so that the time to its occurrence is greater than the time of occurrence of *short-latency reflexes*. See also *long-loop reflex*.

long-loop reflex A *reflex* thought to have a circuit that extends above the spinal segment of the sensory input and motor output. May involve the cerebral cortex. Should be differentiated from reflexes arising from stimulation and recording within a single or adjacent spinal segments (i.e., a segmental reflex). See also *long-latency reflex*.

M response See preferred term, *M wave*.

M wave A *compound muscle action potential* evoked from a muscle by an electric *stimulus* to its *motor nerve*. By convention, the M wave elicited by a supramaximal *stimulus* is used for motor *nerve conduction studies*. Ideally, the *recording electrodes* should be placed so that the initial deflection of the *evoked potential* from the *baseline* is negative. Common measurements include *latency, amplitude*, and *duration*. Also referred to as the *motor response*. Normally, the configuration is biphasic and stable with repeated stimuli at slow rates (1 to 5 *Hz*). See *repetitive nerve stimulation*.

macro motor unit action potential The average electric activity of that part of an anatomic *motor unit* that is within the recording range of a *macro-EMG electrode*. Characterized by consistent appearance when the small recording surface of the macro-EMG electrode is positioned to record *action potentials* from one muscle fiber. The following characteristics can be specified quantitatively: 1) maximal peak-to-peak *amplitude*, 2) area contained under the *waveform*, 3) number of *phases*.

macro MUAP Abbreviation for *macro motor unit action potential*.

macroelectromyography (macro-EMG) General term referring to the technique and conditions that approximate recording of all *muscle fiber action potentials* arising from the same *motor unit*. See *macro motor unit action potential*.

macro-EMG Abbreviation for *macroelectromyography.*

macro-EMG needle electrode A modified *single fiber electromyography* electrode insulated to within 15 mm from the tip and with a small recording surface (25 μm in diameter) 7.5 mm from the tip.

malignant fasciculation Used to describe large, polyphasic *fasciculation potentials* firing at a slow rate. This pattern has been seen in progressive *motor neuron disease,* but the relationship is not exclusive. Use of this term is discouraged. See *fasciculation potential.*

maximal stimulus See *stimulus.*

maximum conduction velocity See *conduction velocity.*

MCD Abbreviation for *mean consecutive difference.* See *jitter.*

mean consecutive difference (MCD) See *jitter.*

mean sorted difference (MSD) See *jitter.*

membrane instability Tendency of a cell membrane to depolarize spontaneously in response to mechanical irritation or following voluntary *activation.* May be used to describe the occurrence of spontaneous single *muscle fiber action potentials* such as *fibrillation potentials* during *needle electrode* examination.

MEP Abbreviation for *motor evoked potential.*

MEPP Abbreviation for *miniature end-plate potential.*

microneurography The technique of recording peripheral nerve *action potentials* in humans by means of intraneural *electrodes.*

miniature end-plate potential (MEPP) The postsynaptic muscle fiber *potentials* produced through the spontaneous release of individual acetylcholine quanta from the presynaptic axon terminal. As recorded with *monopolar* or *concentric needle electrodes* inserted in the end-plate region, MEPPs are monophasic, negative, short *duration* (less than 5 ms), and generally less than 20 μV in *amplitude.*

minimum conduction velocity The *nerve conduction velocity* measured from slowly conducting nerve fibers. Special techniques are needed to produce this measurement in *motor* or *sensory nerves.*

mixed nerve A nerve composed of both motor and sensory axons.

MNCV Abbreviation for *motor nerve conduction velocity.* See *conduction velocity.*

mononeuritis multiplex A disorder characterized by axonal injury and/or *demyelination* affecting nerve fibers in multiple nerves (multiple *mononeuropathies*). Usually occurs in an asymmetric anatomic distribution and in a temporal sequence that is not patterned or symmetric.

mononeuropathy multiplex A disorder characterized by axonal injury and/or *demyelination* affecting nerve fibers exclusively along the course of one named nerve.

monophasic action potential An *action potential* with the *waveform* entirely on one side of the *baseline.*

monophasic end-plate activity See *end-plate activity (monophasic).*

monopolar needle electrode A solid wire *electrode* coated with Teflon^{TM}, except at the tip. Despite the term monopolar, a separate surface or subcutaneous reference electrode is required for recording electric signals. May also be used as a *cathode* in *nerve conduction studies* with another electrode serving as an *anode.*

motor evoked potential (MEP) A *compound muscle action potential* produced by either *transcranial magnetic stimulation* or *transcranial electrical stimulation.*

motor latency Interval between the onset of a *stimulus* and the onset of the resultant *compound muscle action potential (M wave).* The term may be qualified, as proximal motor latency or *distal motor latency,* depending on the relative position of the stimulus.

motor nerve A nerve containing axons which innervate extrafusal and intrafusal muscle fibers. These nerves also contain sensory afferent fibers from muscle and other deep structures.

motor nerve conduction velocity (MNCV) The speed of propagation of *action potentials* along a *motor nerve.* See *conduction velocity.*

motor neuron disease A clinical condition characterized by degeneration of *motor nerve* cells in the brain, brainstem, and spinal cord. The location of degeneration determines the clinical presentation. Primary lateral sclerosis occurs when degeneration affects mainly corticospinal tract motor fibers. Spinal muscular atrophy occurs when degeneration affects lower motor neurons. Amyotrophic lateral sclerosis occurs when degeneration affects both corticospinal tracts and lower motor neurons.

motor point The site over a muscle where its *contraction* may be elicited by a minimal intensity short *duration* electric *stimulus.*

motor response 1) The *compound muscle action potential (M wave)* recorded over a muscle in response to stimulation of the nerve to the muscle. 2) The muscle twitch or *contraction* elicited by stimulation of the nerve to a muscle. 3) The muscle twitch elicited by the *muscle stretch reflex.*

motor unit The anatomic element consisting of an anterior horn cell, its axon, the neuromuscular junctions, and all of the muscle fibers innervated by the axon.

motor unit action potential (MUAP) The *compound action potential* of a single *motor unit* whose muscle fibers lie within the recording range of an *electrode.* With voluntary muscle *contraction,* it is characterized by its consistent appearance and relationship to the force of the contraction. The following measures may be specified, quantitatively if possible, after the *recording electrode* is placed randomly within the muscle:
1. Configuration
    a. *Amplitude,* peak-to-peak (μV or mV).
    b. *Duration,* total (ms).
    c. Number of *phases* (monophasic, biphasic, triphasic, tetraphasic, polyphasic).
    d. Polarity of each phase (negative, positive).
    e. Number of *turns.*
    f. Variation of shape *(jiggle),* if any, with consecutive *discharges.*
    g. Presence of *(satellite linked) potentials,* if any.
    h. *Spike* duration, including satellites.
2. *Recruitment* characteristics
    a. *Threshold* of *activation* (first recruited, low threshold, high threshold).
    b. *Onset frequency.*
    c. *Recruitment frequency (Hz)* or *recruitment interval* (ms) of individual potentials.

Descriptive terms implying diagnostic significance are not recommended, e.g., *myopathic, neuropathic, regeneration, nascent, giant, BSAP* and *BSAPP.* See *polyphasic action potential, serrated action potential.*

motor unit fraction See *scanning EMG.*

motor unit number counting See the preferred term *motor unit number estimate (MUNE).*

motor unit number estimate (MUNE) A quantitative technique for determining the number of functioning *motor units* in a muscle. A variety of methods, including *spike*-triggered *averaging,* incremental *motor nerve* stimulation, *F-wave* measurement, and a Poisson statistical technique can be used. Synonyms can include *motor unit number estimation* and *motor unit number estimating.*

motor unit number estimating (MUNE) See *motor unit number estimate (MUNE).*

motor unit number estimation (MUNE) See *motor unit number estimate (MUNE).*

motor unit potential (MUP) See synonym, *motor unit action potential.*

motor unit territory The area of a muscle cross-section within which the muscle fibers belonging to an individual *motor unit* are distributed.

movement artifact See *artifact.*

movement-related cortical potential Electroencephalogram activity associated with (before and after) a voluntary movement. There are several components including the *Bereitschaftspotential* before the movement and the motor potential at about the time of the movement. See also *Bereitschaftspotential.*

MSD Abbreviation for *mean sorted difference.* See *jitter.*

MUAP Abbreviation for *motor unit action potential.*

multi MUP analysis A *template matching, decomposition EMG* method used for *MUAP* analysis.

multielectrode See *multilead electrode.*

multifocal motor neuropathy A disease characterized by selective focal block of *motor nerve* conduction in multiple nerves. Motor *nerve conduction studies* may permit identification and localization of the segments of nerve affected by the underlying pathology.

multilead electrode Three or more insulated wires inserted through apertures in a common metal cannula with their bared tips flush with the cannula's outer circumference. The arrangement of the bare tips relative to the axis of the cannula and the distance between each tip should be specified. See *electrode.*

multiple discharge Four or more *motor unit action potentials* of the same form and nearly the same *amplitude* occurring consistently in the same relationship to one another and generated by the same axon. See *double* and *triple discharge*.

multiplet See *multiple discharge*.

MUNE Abbreviation for *motor unit number estimate, motor unit number estimation,* and *motor unit number estimating*.

MUP Abbreviation for *motor unit potential*. See preferred term, *motor unit action potential*.

muscle action potential Term commonly used to refer to a *compound muscle action potential*.

muscle atrophy Decrease in size of a muscle that may be due to disease of nerve or muscle, or to disuse.

muscle cramp An involuntary, painful muscle *contraction* associated with electrical activity. *Cramp discharges* are most common, but other types of *repetitive discharges* can also be seen.

muscle fiber action potential *Action potential* recorded from a single muscle fiber.

muscle fiber conduction velocity The speed of propagation of a single *muscle fiber action potential*, usually expressed as meters per second. Usually less than most *nerve conduction velocities*, varies with the rate of *discharge* of the muscle fiber, and requires special techniques for measurement.

muscle hypertrophy Increase in the size of a muscle due to an increase in the size of the muscle fibers or replacement or displacement of muscle fibers by other tissues. The latter is also referred to by the term *pseudo-hypertrophy*, because the muscle is enlarged but weak. Muscle fibers increase in size as a physiologic *response* to repetitive and forceful voluntary *contraction* or as a pathologic response to involuntary electric activity in a muscle, for example, *myotonic discharges* or *complex repetitive discharges*.

muscle stretch reflex *Activation* of a muscle that follows stretch of the muscle, e.g. by percussion of a muscle tendon. See *stretch reflex, T wave*.

muscle tone See *tone*.

myasthenia gravis A disease characterized by muscle weakness that increases with repetitive muscle *activation*. Most commonly, an autoimmune disease caused by the presence of antibodies to the acetylcholine receptors at the neuromuscular junction.

myoclonus A quick jerk of a body part produced by a brief muscle *contraction* typi-cally originating from activity in the central nervous system. Based on the anatomic location of the pathology, may be classified as spinal, segmental, brainstem, or cortical.

myoedema Focal muscle *contraction* produced by muscle percussion. Not associated with propagated electric activity. May be seen in hypothyroidism (myxedema) and chronic malnutrition.

myokymia Continuous quivering or undulating movement of surface and overlying skin and mucous membrane associated with spontaneous, *repetitive discharge* of *motor unit action potentials*. See *myokymic discharge, fasciculation,* and *fasciculation potential*.

myokymic discharge A form of *involuntary activity* in which *motor unit action potentials* fire repetitively and may be associated with clinical *myokymia*. Two firing patterns have been described: 1) Commonly, the *discharge* is a brief, repetitive firing of single motor unit action potentials for a short period (up to a few seconds) at a uniform rate (2 to 60 *Hz*) followed by a short period (up to a few seconds) of silence, with repetition of the same sequence for a particular potential at regular intervals. 2) Rarely, the potential recurs continuously at a fairly uniform *firing rate* (1 to 5 Hz). Myokymic discharges are a subclass of *grouped discharges* and *repetitive discharges*. See also *ephapse* and *ephaptic transmission*.

myopathic motor unit potential Low *amplitude*, short *duration*, polyphasic *motor unit action potentials*. Use of term discouraged. It incorrectly implies specific diagnostic significance of a motor unit action potential configuration. See *motor unit action potential*.

myopathic recruitment Used to describe an increase in the number and *firing rate* of *motor unit action potentials* compared with normal for the strength of muscle *contraction*. Use of term discouraged.

myopathy Disorder affecting the structure and/or function of muscle fibers. Etiologies include hereditary, congenital, mitochondrial, inflammatory, metabolic, infectious, neoplastic, vascular, and traumatic diseases. Most, but not all of these disorders, show abnormalities on needle *electromyography*.

myotonia Delayed relaxation of a muscle after voluntary *contraction* or percussion.

Associated with propagated electric activity, such as *myotonic discharges, complex repetitive discharges* or *neuromyotonic discharges.*

myotonic discharge *Repetitive discharge* that occurs at rates of 20 to 80 *Hz.* There are two types: 1) Biphasic (positive-negative) *spike potentials* less that 5 ms in *duration* resembling *fibrillation potentials.* 2) *Positive waves* of 5 to 20 ms duration resembling *positive sharp waves.* Both potential forms are recorded after *needle electrode* insertion, after voluntary muscle *contraction* or after muscle percussion, and are due to independent, repetitive discharges of single muscle fibers. The *amplitude* and *frequency* of the potentials must both wax and wane. This change produces a characteristic musical sound in the audio output of the *electromyograph* due to the corresponding change in pitch, which has been likened to the sound of a "dive bomber." Contrast with *waning discharge.*

myotonic potential See preferred term, *myotonic discharge.*

NAP Abbreviation for *nerve action potential.* See *compound nerve action potential.*

nascent motor unit potential From the Latin *nascens,* "to be born." Refers to very low *amplitude,* short *duration,* highly polyphasic *motor unit action potentials* observed during early states of reinnervation. Use of term is discouraged, as it incorrectly implies diagnostic significance of a motor unit action potential configuration. See *motor unit action potential.*

NCS Abbreviation for *nerve conduction study.*

NCV Abbreviation for *nerve conduction velocity.* See *conduction velocity.*

near-field A region of electrical activity where the isopotential *voltage* lines associated with a current source change rapidly over a short distance. The terms near-field and *far-field* are arbitrary designations, as there are no agreed-upon criteria defining where the near-field ends and the far-field begins. Compare with *far-field.*

needle electrode An electrical device used for recording or stimulating that is positioned near the tissue of interest by penetration of the skin. See specific electrodes: *bifilar (bipolar) needle recording electrode, concentric needle electrode, macro-EMG needle electrode, monopolar needle electrode, multilead electrode, single fiber needle electrode, and stimulating electrode.*

nerve action potential (NAP) Strictly defined, refers to an *action potential* recorded from a single nerve fiber. The term is commonly used to refer to the *compound nerve action potential.* See *compound nerve action potential.*

nerve conduction study (NCS) Recording and analysis of electric *waveforms* of biologic origin elicited in response to electric or physiologic *stimuli.* The waveforms are *compound sensory nerve action potentials, compound muscle action potentials,* or *mixed nerve action potentials.* The compound muscle action potentials are generally referred to by letters that have historical origin: *M wave, F wave, H wave, T wave, A wave, and R1, R2 waves.* It is possible under standardized conditions to establish normal ranges for *amplitude, duration,* and *latency* of the waveforms and to calculate the maximum *conduction velocity* of *sensory* and *motor* nerves. The term generally refers to studies of waveforms generated in the peripheral nervous system, whereas *evoked potential studies* refers to studies of waveforms generated in both the peripheral and central nervous systems. Synonymous with *electroneurography.*

nerve conduction velocity (NCV) The speed of *action potential* propagation along a nerve fiber or nerve trunk. Generally assumed to refer to the maximum speed of propagation unless otherwise specified. See *conduction velocity.*

nerve fiber action potential *Action potential* recorded from a single axon.

nerve potential Equivalent to *nerve action potential.* Also commonly, but inaccurately, used to refer to the biphasic form of *end-plate activity* observed during *needle electrode* examination of muscle. The latter use is incorrect, because muscle fibers, not nerve fibers, are the source of these *potentials.*

nerve trunk action potential See preferred term, *compound nerve action potential.*

neurapraxia Clinical term used to describe the reversible motor and sensory deficits produced by focal compressive or traction lesions of large myelinated nerve fibers. It is due to *conduction block,* most often caused by focal *demyelination,* but, when very short lived, presumably caused by focal ischemia. The axon is not injured at the lesion site. Compare with *axonotmesis* and *neurotmesis.*

neuromuscular transmission disorder Clinical disorder associated with pathology affecting the structure and function of the neuromuscular junction and interfering with synaptic transmission at that site. Specific diseases include *myasthenia gravis*, Lambert-Eaton myasthenic syndrome, and botulism.

neuromyopathy Clinical disorder associated with pathology affecting both nerve and muscle fibers.

neuromyotonia Clinical syndrome of continuous muscle fiber activity manifested as continuous muscle rippling and stiffness. It may be associated with delayed relaxation following voluntary muscle *contraction*. The accompanying electric activity may be intermittent or continuous. Terms used to describe related clinical syndromes are continuous muscle fiber activity syndrome, Isaac syndrome, Isaac-Merton syndrome, quantal squander syndrome, generalized *myokymia*, pseudomyotonia, normocalcemic *tetany* and neurotonia. Distinguish from *myotonia*.

neuromyotonic discharge Bursts of *motor unit action potentials* that fire at high rates (150 to 300 *Hz*) for a few seconds, often starting or stopping abruptly. The *amplitude* of the *waveforms* typically wanes. *Discharges* may occur spontaneously or be initiated by *needle electrode* movement, voluntary effort, ischemia, or percussion of a nerve. The activity originates in motor axons. Distinguish from *myotonic discharges* and *complex repetitive discharges*. One type of electrical activity recorded in patients who have clinical *neuromyotonia*.

neuropathic motor unit potential Abnormally high-*amplitude*, long-*duration*, polyphasic *motor unit action potential*. Use of term discouraged. Incorrectly implies a specific diagnostic significance of a motor unit action potential configuration. See *motor unit action potential*.

neuropathic recruitment A *recruitment* pattern characterized by a decreased number of *motor unit action potentials* firing at a rapid rate. Use of term discouraged. See preferred terms, *reduced interference pattern, discrete activity, single unit pattern*.

neuropathy Disorder of the peripheral nerves. May be classified by the anatomical structure of the nerve most affected by the disease: cell body (neuronopathy), the axon (axonopathy), or the myelin sheath (demyelinating neuropathy). May selectively affect *motor* or *sensory nerves* or both simultaneously. The etiology may be hereditary, metabolic, inflammatory, toxic, or unknown.

neurotmesis Partial or complete nerve severance including the axons, associated myelin sheaths, and supporting connective tissues, resulting in *axonal degeneration* distal to the injury site. Compare with *axonotmesis, neurapraxia*.

neurotonic discharges Repetitive *motor unit action potentials* recorded from intramuscular *electrodes* during *intraoperative monitoring*. Thought to arise from irritation or injury of nerves supplying the muscle from which the recording is made.

noise Electric activity not related to the signal of interest. In *electrodiagnostic medicine*, *waveforms* generated by *electrodes*, cables, amplifier, or storage media and unrelated to potentials of biologic origin. The term has also been used loosely to refer to one form of *end-plate activity*.

onset frequency The lowest stable *firing rate* for a single *motor unit action potential* that can be voluntarily maintained by a subject.

order of activation The sequence of appearance of different *motor unit action potentials* with increasing strength of voluntary *contraction*. See *recruitment*.

orthodromic Propagation of a nerve impulse in the same direction as physiologic conduction; e.g., conduction along *motor nerve* fibers toward the muscle and conduction along *sensory nerve* fibers towards the spinal cord. Contrast with *antidromic*.

paired stimuli Two consecutive stimuli delivered in a time-locked fashion. The time interval between the two stimuli and the intensity of each *stimulus* can be varied but should be specified. The first stimulus is called the *conditioning stimulus* and the second stimulus is the *test stimulus*. The conditioning stimulus may modify tissue *excitability*, which is then evaluated by the *response* to the test stimulus.

parasite potential See preferred term, *satellite potential*.

peak latency Interval between the onset of a *stimulus* and a specified peak of an evoked *waveform*.

peroneal neuropathy at the knee A *mononeuropathy* involving the common peroneal nerve as it passes around the head of the fibula. The presumed mechanism is compression of the nerve against the fibula. See also *crossed leg palsy*.

phase That portion of a *waveform* between the departure from, and the return to, the *baseline*.

plexopathy Axonal and/or demyelinating disorder affecting the nerve fibers exclusive to the cervical, brachial, lumbar, or sacral rearrangement of spinal nerve roots into peripheral nerves.

polarization The presence of an electric *potential* difference usually across an excitable cell membrane.

polyneuropathy Axonal and/or demyelinating disorder affecting nerve fibers, usually in a symmetrical fashion. The distal segments of the longer nerves in the lower extremities are usually the most severely affected. May be classified as sensory, motor, or sensorimotor depending on the function of nerve fibers affected.

polyphasic action potential An *action potential* with four or more *baseline* crossings, producing five or more *phases*. See *phase*. Contrast with *serrated action potential*.

polyradiculoneuropathy See *radiculopathy*.

positive sharp wave A biphasic, positive then negative *action potential* of a single muscle fiber. It is initiated by *needle electrode* movement (insertional or unsustained positive sharp wave) or occurs spontaneously. Typically *discharge* in a uniform, regular pattern at a rate of 1 to 50 *Hz*; the discharge *frequency* may decrease slightly just before cessation of discharge. The initial positive deflection is rapid (<1 ms), its *duration* is usually less than 5 ms, and the *amplitude* is up to 1 mV. The negative *phase* is of low amplitude, and its duration is 10 to 100 ms. A sequence of positive sharp waves is commonly referred to as a *train of positive sharp waves*. Assumed to be recorded from a damaged area of a muscle fiber. This configuration may result from the position of the needle electrode, which is believed to be adjacent to the depolarized segment of a muscle fiber injured by the electrode. Note that the positive sharp *waveform* is not specific for muscle fiber damage. May occur in association with *fibrillation potentials* and are thought by some to be equivalent discharges. *Motor unit action potentials* and potentials in *myotonic discharges* may have the configuration of positive sharp waves.

positive wave Loosely defined, the term refers to a *positive sharp wave*. See preferred term *positive sharp wave*.

postactivation The period following voluntary *activation* of a nerve or muscle. Contrast with *posttetanic*.

postactivation depression A reduction in the *amplitude* and area of the *M wave(s)* in response to a single *stimulus* or *train of stimuli*, which occurs within a few minutes following a 10- to 60-second strong voluntary *contraction*. *Postactivation exhaustion* refers to the cellular mechanisms responsible for the observed phenomenon of postactivation depression. Also used to describe reduction of the M wave following a *tetanus*, which more logically should be termed *posttetanic depression*.

postactivation exhaustion A reduction in the safety factor (margin) of neuromuscular transmission after sustained *activation* at the neuromuscular junction. The changes in the configuration of the *M wave* due to postactivation exhaustion are referred to as *postactivation depression*.

postactivation facilitation See *facilitation*.

postactivation potentiation An increase in the force of *contraction* (mechanical *response*) after a strong voluntary contraction. Contrast *postactivation facilitation*.

posttetanic The period following *tetanus*. Contrast with *postactivation*.

posttetanic depression See *postactivation depression*.

posttetanic facilitation See *facilitation, potentiation*.

posttetanic potentiation 1) The incrementing mechanical *response* of muscle during and after *repetitive nerve stimulation*. 2) In central nervous system physiology, enhancement of *excitability* or *reflex* outflow of neuronal systems following a long period of high-*frequency* stimulation. See *facilitation, potentiation*.

potential 1) A difference in charges, measurable in volts, that exists between two points. Most biologically produced potentials arise from the difference in charge between two sides of a cell membrane. 2) A term for a physiologically recorded *waveform*.

potentiation Physiologically, the enhancement of a *response*. The convention used in this glossary is to use the term *potentiation* to describe the incrementing mechanical response of muscle elicited by *repetitive nerve stimulation*, e.g., *posttetanic potentiation*, whereas the term *facilitation* is used to describe the incrementing electrical response elicited by *repetitive nerve stimulation*, e.g., *postactivation facilitation*.

prolonged insertion activity See *insertion activity*.

propagation velocity of a muscle fiber The speed of transmission of a *muscle fiber action potential*.

pseudodecrement An *artifact* produced by movement of the *stimulating* or *recording electrodes* during *repetitive nerve stimulation*. The *amplitude* and area of the *M wave* can vary in a way that resembles a *decrementing response*; however, the *responses* are generally irregular and not reproducible.

pseudofacilitation See *facilitation*.

pseudohypertrophy See *muscle hypertrophy*.

pseudomyotonic discharge Formerly used to describe *complex repetitive discharges*. Use of term discouraged.

pseudopolyphasic action potential Use of term discouraged. See preferred term, *serrated action potential*.

QEMG Abbreviation for *quantitative electromyography*.

QSART Abbreviation for *quantitative sudomotor axon reflex test*.

QST Abbreviation for *quantitative sensory testing*.

quantitative electromyography (QEMG) A systematic method for measuring the recordings made by an intramuscular *needle electrode*. Measurements include *motor unit action potential* characteristics such as *amplitude, duration*, and *phases*, or *interference pattern* characteristics. See *turns* and *amplitude analysis*.

quantitative sensory testing (QST) An instrumented method for measuring cutaneous sensation.

quantitative sudomotor axon reflex test (QSART) Test of postganglionic sympathetic sudomotor axon function by measuring sweat output following *activation* of axon terminals by local application of acetylcholine. *Antidromic* transmission of the impulse from the nerve terminals reaches a branch point, then travels *orthodromically* to release acetylcholine from the nerve terminals, inducing a sweating *response*. In small fiber *polyneuropathy*, the response may be reduced or absent. In

painful *neuropathies*, and in *reflex* sympathetic dystrophy, the response may be excessive and persistent or reduced.

R1, R2 waves See *blink responses*.

radiculopathy Axonal and/or demyelinating disorder affecting the nerve fibers exclusive to one spinal nerve root or spinal nerve. May affect the anterior (motor) or posterior (sensory) spinal nerve roots, or both, at one spinal cord segment level. The resulting clinical syndrome may include pain, sensory loss, parethesia, weakness, *fasciculations*, and *muscle atrophy*. If more than one spinal root is involved, the term *polyradiculopathy* may be used as a descriptor.

raster A method for display of a free-running sweep in *electromyography*. Sweeps are offset vertically so that each successive sweep is displayed below the one preceding it.

raw EMG Unprocessed *EMG* signal recorded with surface or intramuscular *electrodes*.

reciprocal inhibition Inhibition of a motor neuron pool secondary to the *activation* of the motor neuron pool of its antagonist. It is one of several important spinal mechanisms of motor control that help to make movements smoother and utilize less energy. There are multiple mechanisms for reciprocal inhibition, including one mediated by the Ia inhibitory interneuron that activates Ia afferents and disynaptically inhibits the muscle that is antagonist to the source of the Ia afferents.

recording electrode Device used to record electric *potential* difference. All electric recordings require two *electrodes*. The electrode close to the source of the activity to be recorded is called the *active* or *exploring electrode*, and the other recording electrode is called the *reference electrode*. Active electrode is synonymous with *input terminal 1*, or *E-1* (or older terms whose use is discouraged, *grid 1*, and *G1*). Reference electrode is synonymous with *input terminal 2*, or *E-2* (or older terms whose use is discouraged *grid 2*, and *G2*). In some recordings it is not certain which electrode is closer to the source of the biologic activity, e.g. recording with a *bifilar needle recording electrode*, or when attempting to define *far-field* potentials. In this situation, it is convenient to refer to one electrode as input electrode 1, or E-1, and the other as input electrode 2, or E-2. By present convention, a potential difference that is negative at the active electrode (input terminal 1, E-1) relative to the reference electrode (input terminal 2, E-2) causes an upward deflection on the display screen. The term "monopolar recording" is not recommended, because all recordings require two electrodes; however, it is commonly used to describe the use of one type of intramuscular *needle electrode*. A similar combination of needle electrodes has been used to record nerve activity and also has been referred to as "monopolar recording."

recruitment The successive *activation* of the same and additional *motor units* with increasing strength of voluntary muscle *contraction*. See *motor unit action potential*.

recruitment frequency *Firing rate* of a *motor unit action potential (MUAP)* when a different MUAP first appears during gradually increasing voluntary muscle *contraction*. This parameter is essential to assessment of *recruitment pattern*.

recruitment interval The *interdischarge interval* between two consecutive *discharges* of a *motor unit action potential (MUAP)* when a different MUAP first appears during gradually increasing voluntary muscle *contraction*. The reciprocal of the recruitment interval is the *recruitment frequency*. See also *interdischarge interval*.

recruitment pattern A qualitative and/or quantitative description of the sequence of appearance of *motor unit action potentials* during increasing voluntary muscle *contraction*. The *recruitment frequency* and *recruitment interval* are two quantitative measures commonly used. See *interference pattern, early recruitment, reduced recruitment* for qualitative terms commonly used.

recurrent inhibition Decreased probability of firing of a motor neuron pool mediated by Renshaw cells. Renshaw cells are activated by recurrent collaterals from the axons of alpha-motoneurons. Such inhibition influences the same cells that originate the excitatory impulses and their neighbors.

reduced insertion activity See *insertion activity*.

reduced interference pattern See *interference pattern*.

reduced recruitment pattern A descriptive term for the *interference pattern* when the number of *motor units* available to generate a muscle *contraction* are reduced. One cause for a *reduced interference pattern*. See *interference pattern, recruitment pattern*.

reference electrode See *recording electrode*.

reflex A stereotyped *motor response* elicited by a sensory *stimulus* and a *response*. Its anatomic pathway consists of an afferent, *sensory* input to the central nervous system, at least one synaptic connection, and an efferent output to an effector organ. The response is most commonly *motor*, but reflexes involving autonomic effector organs also occur. Examples include the *H reflex* and the sudomotor reflex. See *H wave, quantitative sudomotor axon reflex test*.

refractory period General term for the time following an *action potential* when an excitable membrane cannot be stimulated to produce another action potential. The *absolute refractory period* is the time following an action potential during which no *stimulus*, however strong, evokes a further *response*. The *relative refractory period* is the time following an action potential during which a stimulus must be abnormally large to evoke a second response. The *functional refractory period* is the time following an action potential during which a second action potential cannot yet excite the given region.

refractory period of transmission Interval following an *action potential* during which a nerve cannot conduct a second one. Distinguish from *refractory period*, as commonly used, which deals with the ability of a *stimulus* to produce an action potential.

regeneration motor unit potential Use of term discouraged. See *motor unit action potential*.

relative refractory period See *refractory period*.

repair of the decrement See *facilitation*.

repetitive discharge General term for the recurrence of an *action potential* with the same or nearly identical form. May refer to recurring potentials recorded in muscle at rest, during voluntary *contraction*, or in response to a single nerve *stimulus*. See *double discharge, triple discharge, multiple discharge, myokymic discharge, complex repetitive discharge, neuromyotonic discharge,* and *cramp discharge*.

repetitive nerve stimulation The technique of repeated *supramaximal stimulation* of a nerve while recording successive *M waves* from a muscle innervated by the nerve. Commonly used to assess the integrity of neuromuscular transmission.

The number of *stimuli* and the *frequency* of stimulation should be specified. *Activation procedures* performed as a part of the test should be specified, e.g., sustained voluntary *contraction* or contraction induced by nerve stimulation. If the test includes an activation procedure, the time elapsed after its completion should also be specified. For a description of specific patterns of *responses*, see *incrementing response, decrementing response, facilitation,* and *postactivation depression.*

repolarization A return in membrane *potential* from a depolarized state toward the normal resting level.

residual latency The calculated time difference between the measured *distal latency* of a *motor nerve* and the expected latency, calculated by dividing the distance between the stimulating *cathode* and the active *recording electrode* by the maximum *conduction velocity* measured in a more proximal segment of the nerve. It is due in part to neuromuscular transmission time and to slowing of conduction velocity in terminal axons due to decreasing diameter and the presence of unmyeliated segments.

response An activity elicited by a *stimulus.*

resting membrane potential *Voltage* across the membrane of an excitable cell in the absence of a *stimulus.* See *polarization.*

rheobase See *strength-duration curve.*

rigidity A velocity independent increase in *muscle tone* and stiffness with full range of joint motion as interpreted by the clinical examiner from the physical examination. Often associated with simultaneous low-grade *contraction* of agonist and antagonist muscles. Like muscle *spasticity,* the involuntary *motor unit action potential* activity increases with activity or passive stretch. Does not seem to change with the velocity of stretch, and, on passive stretch, the increased tone has a "lead pipe" or constant quality. It is a cardinal feature of central nervous system disorders affecting the basal ganglia. Contrast with *spasticity.*

rise time The interval from the onset of a polarity change of a *potential* to its peak. The method of measurement should be specified.

satellite potential A small *action potential* separated from the main *motor unit action potential* by an isoelectric interval that fires in a time-locked relationship to the main action potential. It usually follows, but may precede, the main action potential. Less preferred terms include *late component, parasite potential, linked potential,* and *coupled discharge.*

scanning EMG A technique by which a *needle electrode* is advanced in defined steps through muscle while a separate *SFEMG* electrode is used to trigger both the display sweep and the advancement device. Provides temporal and spatial information about the *motor unit.* Distinct maxima in the recorded activity are considered to be generated by muscle fibers innervated by a common branch of an axon. These groups of fibers form a *motor unit fraction.*

sea shell sound (sea shell roar or noise) Use of term discouraged. See *end-plate activity, monophasic.*

sensory latency Interval between the onset of a *stimulus* and the onset of the negative deflection of the *compound sensory nerve action potential.* This term has been used loosely to refer to the *sensory peak latency.* May be qualified as proximal sensory latency or distal sensory latency, depending on the relative position of the stimulus.

sensory nerve A nerve containing only sensory fibers, composed mainly of axons innervating cutaneous receptors.

sensory nerve action potential (SNAP) See *compound sensory nerve action potential.*

sensory nerve conduction velocity The speed of propagation of *action potentials* along a *sensory nerve.*

sensory peak latency Interval between the onset of a *stimulus* and the peak of the negative *phase* of the *compound sensory nerve action potential.* Contrast with *sensory latency.*

sensory potential Synonym for the more precise term, *compound sensory nerve action potential.*

sensory response Synonym for the more precise term, *compound sensory nerve action potential.*

SEP Abbreviation for *somatosensory evoked potential.*

serrated action potential A *waveform* with several changes in direction *(turns)* that do not cross the *baseline.* Most often used to describe a *motor unit action potential.* The term is preferred to *complex motor unit action potential* and *pseudopolyphasic action potential.* See also *turn* and *polyphasic action potential.*

SFEMG Abbreviation for *single fiber electro-myography*.

shock artifact See *artifact*.

short-latency reflex A *reflex* with one (monosynaptic) or few (oligosynaptic) synapses. Used in contrast to *long-latency reflex*.

short-latency somatosensory evoked potential (SSEP) That portion of the *waveforms* of a *somatosensory evoked potential* normally occurring within 25 ms after stimulation of the median nerve in the upper extremity at the wrist, 40 ms after stimulation of the common peroneal nerve in the lower extremity at the knee, and 50 ms after stimulation of the posterior tibial nerve at the ankle.

signal averager A digital device that improves the signal-to-*noise* ratio of an electrophysiological recording by adding successive time-locked recordings to preceding traces and computing the average value of each data point. A signal acquired by this method is described as an "averaged" *waveform*.

silent period A pause in the electric activity of a muscle that may be produced by many different *stimuli*. Stimuli used commonly in clinical neurophysiology include rapid unloading of a muscle, electrical stimulation of a peripheral nerve or *transcranial magnetic stimulation*.

single fiber electromyography (SFEMG) The technique and conditions that permit recording of single *muscle fiber action potentials*. See *single fiber needle electrode, blocking,* and *jitter*.

single fiber EMG See *single fiber electromyography*.

single fiber needle electrode A *needle electrode* with a small recording surface (usually 25 μm in diameter), which permits the recording of single *muscle fiber action potentials* between the recording surface and the cannula. See *single fiber electromyography*.

single unit pattern See *interference pattern*.

SNAP Abbreviation for *sensory nerve action potential*. See *compound sensory nerve action potential*.

snap, crackle, and pop A benign type of *increased insertion activity* that follows, after a very brief period of electrical silence, the normal *insertion activity* generated by *needle electrode* movement. It consists of trains of *potentials* that vary in length; how-ever, they can persist for a few seconds. Each train consists of a series of up to 10 or more potentials in which the individual components fire at irregular intervals. The potentials consistently vary in *amplitude, duration,* and configuration. Individual potentials may be mono-, bi-, tri-, or multiphasic in appearance; they often have a positive *waveform*. The variation on sequential firings produces a distinctive sound, hence the name. Seen most often in those with mesomorphic builds, especially young adult males. Found most often in lower extremity muscles, especially the medial gastrocnemius.

somatosensory evoked potential (SEP) Electric *wave-forms* of biologic origin elicited by electric stimulation or physiologic *activation* of peripheral *sensory nerves* and recorded from peripheral and central nervous system structures. Normally is a complex *waveform* with several components, which are specified by polarity and average *peak latency*. The polarity and latency of individual components depend upon 1) subject variables, such as age, gender, and body habitus, 2) *stimulus* characteristics, such as intensity and rate of stimulation, and 3) recording parameters, such as amplifier time constants, *electrode* placement, and electrode combinations. See *short-latency somatosensory evoked potentials*.

spasticity A velocity-dependent increase in *muscle tone* due to a disease process that interrupts the suprasegmental tracts to the alpha motor neurons, gamma motor neurons, or segmental spinal neurons. May be elicited and interpreted by the clinical examiner during the physical examination by brisk passive movement of a limb at the joint. Almost uniformly accompanied by hyperreflexia, a Babinski sign, and other signs of upper motor neuron pathology, including clonus and the clasp-knife phenomenon. The clasp-knife phenomenon is a rapid decrease of tone following a period of increased tone during passive rotation of the joint. The pathophysiology is not certain and may include more than dysfunction of the corticospinal tracts.

spike 1) A short-lived (1 to 3 ms), all-or-none *waveform* that arises when an excitable membrane reaches *threshold*. 2) The electric record of a nerve or muscle impulse.

spinal evoked potential Electric *waveforms* of biologic origin recorded over the spine in response to electric stimulation or physiologic *activation* of peripheral sensory fibers. See preferred term, *somatosensory evoked potential.*

spontaneous activity Electric activity recorded from muscle at rest after *insertion activity* has subsided and when there is not voluntary *contraction* or an external *stimulus.* Compare with *involuntary activity.*

SSEP Abbreviation for *short-latency somatosensory evoked potential.*

staircase phenomenon The progressive increase in muscle *contraction* force observed in response to continued low rates of muscle *activation.*

startle (reflex) A *response* produced by an unanticipated *stimulus* that leads to alerting and protective movements such as eyelid closure and flexion of the limbs. Auditory stimuli are typically most efficacious.

stiffman syndrome A disorder characterized by continuous muscle *contraction* giving rise to severe stiffness. Axial muscles are typically affected most severely. Patients have difficulty moving. Walking and voluntary movements are slow. Sensory stimulation often induces severe spasms. *Electromyography* demonstrates continuous activity of *motor unit action potentials* in a normal pattern that cannot be silenced by contraction of the antagonist muscle. It is often associated with circulating antibodies to glutamic acid decarboxylase (GAD), and the resulting deficiency of GABA may play a role in its pathophysiology. Since women are affected in equal or greater numbers than men, the term *stiff-person syndrome* may be preferable.

stiffperson syndrome Synonym for *stiffman syndrome.*

stigmatic electrode A term of historic interest. Used by Sherrington for *active* or *exploring electrode.*

stimulated SFEMG See preferred term *stimulation SFEMG.*

stimulating electrode Device used to deliver electric current. All electric stimulation requires two *electrodes*; the negative terminal is termed the *cathode*, and the positive terminal is the *anode*. By convention, the stimulating electrodes are called *bipolar* if they are encased or attached together and are called *monopolar* if they are not. Electric stimulation for *nerve conduction studies* generally requires application of the cathode in the vicinity of the neural tissue to produce *depolarization.*

stimulation single fiber electromyography (stimulation SFEMG) Use of electrical stimulation instead of voluntary *activation* of *motor units* for the analysis of *single fiber electromyography.* The method is used in patients who are unable to produce a steady voluntary muscle *contraction.* The stimulation can be delivered to intramuscular axons, nerve trunks, or muscle fibers.

stimulus Any external agent, state or change that is capable of influencing the activity of a cell, tissue, or organism. In clinical *nerve conduction studies*, an electric stimulus is applied to a nerve. It may be described in absolute terms or with respect to the *evoked potential* of the nerve or muscle. In absolute terms, it is defined by a *duration* (ms), a *waveform* (square, exponential, linear, etc.), and a strength or intensity measured in *voltage* (V) or current (mA). With respect to the evoked potential, the stimulus may be graded as *subthreshold, threshold, submaximal, maximal,* or *supramaximal.* A threshold stimulus is one just sufficient to produce a detectable *response.* Stimuli less than the threshold stimulus are termed subthreshold. The maximal stimulus is the stimulus intensity after which a further increase in intensity causes no increase in the *amplitude* of the evoked potential. Stimuli of intensity below this level but above threshold are submaximal. Stimuli of intensity greater than the maximal stimulus are termed supramaximal. Ordinarily, supramaximal stimuli are used for nerve conduction studies. By convention, an electric stimulus of approximately 20% greater voltage/current than required for the maximal stimulus is used for supramaximal stimulation. The *frequency*, number and duration of a series of stimuli should be specified.

stimulus artifact See *artifact.*

strength-duration curve Graphic presentation of the relationship between the intensity (Y axis) and various *durations* (X axis) of the *threshold* electric *stimulus* of a nerve or muscle. The *rheobase* is the intensity of an electric current of infinite duration necessary to produce a minimal *action potential*. The *chronaxie* is the time required for an electric current twice the rheobase to elicit the first visible action potential. Measurement of the strength-duration curve is not a common practice in modern *electrodiagnostic medicine*.

stretch reflex A *reflex* produced by passive lengthening of a muscle. The principal sensory *stimuli* come from group Ia and group II muscle spindle afferents. It consists of several *phases*. The earliest component is monosynaptic and is also called the myotatic reflex, or tendon reflex. There are also long-*latency* stretch reflexes. See also *muscle stretch reflex, T wave*.

submaximal stimulus See *stimulus*.

subnormal period A time interval that immediately follows the *supernormal period* of nerve, which is characterized by reduced *excitability* compared to the resting state. Its *duration* is variable and is related to the *refractory period*.

subthreshold stimulus See *stimulus*.

supernormal period A time interval that immediately follows the *refractory period* which corresponds to a very brief period of partial *depolarization*. It is characterized by increased nerve *excitability* and is followed by the *subnormal period*.

supraclavicular plexus That portion of the *brachial plexus* that is located superior to the clavicle.

supraclavicular stimulation Percutaneous nerve stimulation at the base of the neck, which activates the upper, middle, and/or lower trunks of the *brachial plexus*. This term is preferred to *Erb's point stimulation*.

supramaximal stimulus See *stimulus*.

surface electrode Conducting device for stimulating or recording placed on the skin surface. The material (metal, fabric, etc.), configuration (disk, ring, etc.), size, and separation should be specified. See *electrode (ground, recording, stimulating)*.

sympathetic skin response Electrical *potential* resulting from electrodermal activity in sweat glands in response to both direct and *reflex* peripheral or sympathetic trunk stimulation of autonomic activity.

synkinesis Involuntary movement made by muscles distant from those activated voluntarily. It is commonly seen during recovery after *facial neuropathy*. It is due to aberrant reinnervation and/or *ephaptic transmission*.

T wave A *compound muscle action potential* evoked from a muscle by rapid stretch of its tendon, as part of the *muscle stretch reflex*.

tardy ulnar palsy A type of *mononeuropathy* involving the ulnar nerve at the elbow. The nerve becomes compressed or entrapped due to deformity of the elbow from a previous injury. See also *cubital tunnel syndrome* and *ulnar neuropathy at the elbow*.

template matching An automated method used in *quantitative electromyography* for selecting *motor unit action potentials* for measurement by extracting only *potentials* that resemble an initially identified potential.

temporal dispersion Relative desynchronization of components of a *compound muscle action potential* due to different rates of conduction of each synchronously evoked component from the stimulation point to the *recording electrode*. It may be due to normal variability in individual axon *conduction velocities*, especially when assessed over a long nerve segment, or to disorders that affect myelination of nerve fibers.

terminal latency Synonymous with preferred term, *distal latency*. See *motor latency* and *sensory latency*.

TES Abbreviation for *transcranial electrical stimulation*.

test stimulus See *paired stimuli*.

tetanic contraction The *contraction* produced in a muscle through repetitive maximal direct or indirect stimulation at a sufficiently high *frequency* to produce a smooth summation of successive maximum twitches. The term may also be applied to maximum voluntary contractions in which the firing frequencies of most or all of the component *motor units* are sufficiently high that successive twitches of individual motor units fuse smoothly. Their combined tensions produce a steady, smooth, maximum contraction of the whole muscle.

tetanus 1) The continuous *contraction* of muscle caused by repetitive stimulation or *discharge* of nerve or muscle. Contrast with *tetany*. 2) A clinical disorder caused by circulating tetanus toxin. Signs and symptoms are caused by loss of inhibition in the central nervous system and are characterized by muscle spasms, hyperreflexia, seizures, respiratory spasms, and paralysis.

tetany A clinical syndrome manifested by muscle twitching, cramps, and carpal and pedal spasm. These clinical signs are manifestations of peripheral and central nervous system nerve irritability from several causes. In these conditions, *repetitive discharges (double discharge, triple discharge, multiple discharge)* occur frequently with voluntary *activation* of *motor unit action potentials* or may appear as *spontaneous activity*. This activity is enhanced by systemic alkalosis or local ischemia.

tetraphasic action potential *Action potential* with three *baseline* crossings, producing four *phases*.

thermography A technique for measuring infrared emission from portions of the body surface. The degree of emission depends upon the amount of heat produced by the region that is studied. Its use in the diagnosis of *radiculopathy*, peripheral nerve injury, and disorders of the autonomic nervous system is controversial.

thermoregulatory sweat test A technique for assessing the integrity of the central and peripheral efferent sympathetic pathways. It consists of measuring the sweat distribution using an indicator powder while applying a controlled heat *stimulus* to raise body temperature sufficient to induce sweating.

thoracic outlet syndrome An *entrapment neuropathy* caused by compression of the neurovascular bundle as it traverses the shoulder region. Compression arises from acquired or congenital anatomic variations in the shoulder region. Symptoms can be related to compression of vascular structures, portions of the *brachial plexus*, or both.

threshold The level at which a clear and abrupt transition occurs from one state to another. The term is generally used to refer to the *voltage* level at which an *action potential* is initiated in a single axon or muscle fiber or a group of axons or muscle fibers.

threshold stimulus See *stimulus*.

tic Clinical term used to describe a sudden, brief, stereotyped, repetitive movement.

When associated with vocalizations, may be the primary manifestation of Tourette syndrome.

tilt table test A test of autonomic function that is performed by measuring blood pressure and heart rate before and a specified period of time after head up tilt. The *duration* of recording and amount of tilt should be specified.

TMS Abbreviation for *transcranial magnetic stimulation*.

tone The resistance to passive stretch of a joint. When the resistance is high, this is called *hypertonia*, and when the resistance is low, this is called *hypotonia*. Two types of hypertonia are *rigidity* and *spasticity*.

train of positive sharp waves See *positive sharp wave*.

train of stimuli A group of *stimuli*. The *duration* of the group or the number of stimuli as well as the stimulation *frequency* should be specified.

transcranial electrical stimulation (TES) Stimulation of the cortex of the brain through the intact skull and scalp by means of a brief, very high *voltage*, electrical *stimulus*. *Activation* is more likely under the *anode* rather than the *cathode*. Because it is painful, this technique has largely been replaced by *transcranial magnetic stimulation*.

transcranial magnetic stimulation (TMS) Stimulation of the cortex of the brain through the intact skull and scalp by means of a brief magnetic *stimulus*. In practice, a brief pulse of strong current is passed through a coil of wire in order to produce a time-varying magnetic field in the order of 1 to 2 Tesla. Contrast with *transcranial electrical stimulation*.

tremor Rhythmical, involuntary oscillatory movement of a body part.

triphasic action potential *Action potential* with two *baseline* crossings, producing three *phases*.

triple discharge Three *motor unit action potentials* of the same form and nearly the same *amplitude*, occurring consistently in the same relationship to one another and generated by the same axon. The interval between the second and third *action potentials* often exceeds that between the first two, and both are usually in the range of 2 to 20 ms. See also *double discharge, multiple discharge*.

triplet Synonym for the preferred term, *triple discharge.*

turn Point of change in polarity of a *waveform* and the magnitude of the *voltage* change following the turning point. It is not necessary that the voltage change pass through the *baseline.* The minimal excursion required to constitute a change should be specified.

turns and amplitude analysis See preferred term *interference pattern analysis.* Refers to the interference pattern analysis developed by Robin Willison in the 1960s.

ulnar neuropathy at the elbow A *mononeuropathy* involving the ulnar nerve in the region of the elbow. At least two sites of *entrapment neuropathy* have been recognized. The nerve may be entrapped or compressed as it passes through the retrocondylar groove at the elbow. Alternatively, it may be entrapped just distal to the elbow as it passes through the cubital tunnel. Anatomic variations or deformities of the elbow may contribute to nerve injury. See also *cubital tunnel syndrome* and *tardy ulnar palsy.*

unipolar needle electrode See synonym, *monopolar needle recording electrode.*

upper motor neuron syndrome A clinical condition resulting from a pathological process affecting descending motor pathways including the corticospinal tract or its cells of origin. Signs and symptoms include weakness, *spasticity*, and slow and clumsy motor performance. On *electromyographic* examination of weak muscles, there is slow *motor unit action potential* firing at maximal effort.

utilization time See preferred term, *latency of activation.*

Valsalva maneuver A forcible exhalation against the closed glottis which creates an abrupt, transient elevation of intrathoracic and intra-abdominal pressure. This results in a characteristic pattern of heart rate and blood pressure changes that can be used to quantify autonomic function. See *Valsalva ratio.*

Valsalva ratio The ratio of the fastest heart rate occurring at the end of a forced exhalation against a closed glottis (*phase* II of the *Valsalva maneuver*), and the slowest heart rate within 30 seconds after the forced exhalation (phase IV). In patients with disorders of the autonomic nervous system, the ratio may be reduced.

VEP Abbreviation for *visual evoked potential.*

VER Abbreviation for *visual evoked response.* See *visual evoked potential.*

visual evoked potential (VEP) Electric *waveforms* of biologic origin recorded over the cerebrum and elicited in response to visual stimuli. They are classified by *stimulus* rate as transient or steady state, and they can be further divided by stimulus presentation mode. The normal transient VEP to checkerboard pattern reversal or shift has a major positive occipital peak at about 100 ms (P100), often preceded by a negative peak (N75). The precise range of normal values for the *latency* and *amplitude* of P100 depends on several factors: 1) subject variables, such as age, gender, and visual acuity; 2) stimulus characteristics, such as type of stimulator, full-field or half-field stimulation, check size, contrast, and luminescence; and 3) recording parameters, such as placement and combination of *recording electrodes.*

visual evoked response (VER) Synonym for preferred term, *visual evoked potential.*

volitional activity Synonymous with *voluntary activity.*

voltage *Potential* difference between two recording sites usually expressed in volts (V) or millivolts (mV).

volume conduction Spread of current from a *potential* source through a conducting medium, such as body tissues.

voluntary activity In *electromyography*, the electric activity recorded from a muscle with consciously controlled *contraction.* The effort made to contract the muscle may be specified relative to that of a corresponding normal muscle, e.g., minimal, moderate, or maximal. If the recording remains isoelectric during the attempted contraction and equipment malfunction has been excluded, it can be concluded that there is no voluntary activity.

wake-up test A procedure used most commonly in spinal surgery. During critical portions of an operation in which the spinal cord is at risk for injury, the level of general anesthesia is allowed to decrease to the point where the patient can respond to commands. The patient is then asked to move hands and feet, and a movement in response to commands indicates the spinal cord is intact. This procedure is used routinely in some centers. *Somatosensory evoked potential* monitoring has supplanted its use in most centers, except sometimes in the situation where they indicate the possibility of spinal cord injury.

wallerian degeneration Degeneration of the segment of an axon distal to nerve injury that destroys its continuity.

waning discharge A *repetitive discharge* that gradually decreases in *frequency* or *amplitude* before cessation. Contrast with *myotonic discharge*.

wave A transient change in *voltage* represented as a line of differing directions over time.

waveform The shape of a *wave*. The term is often used synonymously with *wave*.

wire electrodes Thin wires that are insulated except for the tips, which are bared. The wire is inserted into muscle with a needle. After the needle is withdrawn, the wire remains in place. Wire electrodes are superior to *surface electrodes* for *kinesiologic EMG*, because they are less affected by *cross talk* from adjacent muscles. They also record selectively from the muscle into which they are inserted.

Bibliography

AAEM glossary of terms in clinical electromyography. Section II: Illustrations of selected waveforms. American Association of Electrodiagnostic Medicine 2001.

Bolton CF: AAEM minimonography no. 40: Clinical neurophysiology of the respiratory system. *Muscle & Nerve* 1993;16:809–818.

Botelho SY, Deaterly DF, Austin S, Comroe JH Jr: Evaluation of electromyogram of patients with myasthenia gravis. *AMA Arch Neurol Psychiatry* 1952;67:441–450.

Braddom RL, Johnson EW: Standardization of H reflex and diagnostic use in S1 radiculopathy. *Arch Phys Med Rehabil* 1974;55:161–166.

Buschbacher RM: Ulnar nerve motor conduction to the abductor digiti minimi. *Am J Phys Med Rehabil* 1999;78(Suppl 6):S9–S14.

Butler ET, Johnson EW: Normal conduction velocity in the lateral femoral cutaneous nerve. *Arch Phys Med Rehabil* 1974;55:31–32.

Campagnolo DI, Romello MA, Park YI, Foye PM, DeLisa JA: Technique for studying in the lateral cutaneous nerve of calf. *Muscle & Nerve* 2000;23:1277–1279.

Campbell WW, Pridgeon RM, Sahni KS: Short segment incremental studies in the evaluation of ulnar neuropathy at the elbow. *Muscle & Nerve* 1992;15:1050–1054.

Campbell WW, Ward LC, Swift RR: Nerve conduction velocity varies inversely with height. *Muscle & Nerve* 1981;4:520–530.

Capozzoli NJ: Aseptic technique in needle EMG: Common sense and common practice. *Muscle & Nerve* 1996;18:538.

Cerra D, Johnson EW: Motor conduction velocity in premature infants. *Arch Phys Med Rehabil* 1962;43:160–164.

Chang CW, Lien IN: Comparison of sensory nerve conduction in the palmar cutaneous branch and first digital branch of the median nerve: A new diagnostic method for carpal tunnel syndrome. *Muscle & Nerve* 1991;14:1173–1176.

Checkles NS, Russakov AD, Piero DL: Ulnar nerve conduction velocity: Effect of elbow position on measurement. *Arch Phys Med Rehabil* 1971;52:362–365.

Clawson DR, Cardenas DD: Dorsal nerve of the penis conduction velocity: A new technique. *Muscle & Nerve* 1991;14:845–849.

Craft S, Currier DP, Nelson RM: Motor conduction of the anterior interosseous nerve. *Phys Ther* 1977;57:1143–1145.

de Visser O, Schimsheimer RJ, Hart AAM: The H reflex of the flexor carpi radialis muscle: A study in controls and radiation-induced brachial plexus lesion. *J Neurol Neurosurg Psychiatry* 1984;47:1098–1101.

Devi S, Lovelace RE, Duarte N: Proximal peroneal nerve conduction velocity: Recording from anterior tibial and peroneus brevis muscles. *Ann Neurol* 1977;2:116–119.

Dick HC, Bradley WE, Scott FB, Timm GW: Pudendal sexual reflex. Electrophysiologic investigation. *Urology* 1979;3:376–379.

Dumitru D, Nelson MR: Posterior femoral cutaneous nerve conduction. *Arch Phys Med Rehabil* 1990;71:979–982.

Felice KJ: Acute anterior interosseous neuropathy in a patient with hereditary neuropathy with liability to pressure palsies: a clinical and electromyographic study. *Muscle & Nerve* 1995;18:1329–1331.

Felsenthal G, Brockman PS, Mondell DL, Hilton EB: Proximal forearm ulnar nerve techniques. *Arch Phys Med Rehabil* 1986;67:440–444.

Fu R, DeLisa JA, Kraft GH: Motor conduction latencies through the tarsal tunnel in normal adult subjects: Standard determinations corrected for temperature and distance. *Arch Phys Med Rehabil* 1980;61:243–248.

Gamstorp I: Normal conduction velocity of ulnar, median, and peroneal nerves in infancy, childhood, and adolescence. *Acta Paediatr Scand* 1963;146(Suppl):68–76.

Gassel MM: Source of error in motor nerve conduction studies. *Neurology* 1964;14:825–835.

Goodgold J, Moldaver J: Changes in electromyographic waveforms in relation to variation in type and position of electrode. *Arch Phys Med Rehabil* 1955;36:627–630.

Green RF, Brien M: Accessory nerve latency to the middle and lower trapezius. *Arch Phys Med Rehabil* 1985;66:23–24.

Gold C, Rosenfalck A, Willison RG: Report of the committee on EMG instrumentation: Technical factors in recording electrical activity of muscle and nerve in man. *Electroencephalogr Clin Neurophysiol* 1970;28:399–413.

Gutmann L: Atypical deep peroneal neuropathy in presence of accessory deep peroneal nerve. *J Neurol Neurosurg Psychiatry* 1970;33:453–456.

Halar EM, Delisa JA, Brozovich FV: Nerve conduction velocity: Relationship of skin, subcutaneous, and intramuscular temperature. *Arch Phys Med Rehabil* 1980;61:199–203.

Halar EM, Delisa JA, Brozovich FV: Peroneal nerve conduction velocity: The importance of temperature correction. *Arch Phys Med Rehab* 1981;62:439–443.

Halar EM, DeLisa JA, Soine TL: Nerve conduction studies in upper extremities: Skin temperature corrections. *Arch Phys Med Rehabil* 1983;64:412–416.

Harvey AM, Masland RL: A method for the study of neuromuscular transmission in human subjects. *Bull Johns Hopkins Hosp* 1941;68:81–93.

Izzo KL, Aravabhumi S, Jafri A, Sobel E, Demopoulous JT: Medial and lateral antebrachial cutaneous nerves: Standardization of technique, reliability and age effect on healthy subjects. *Arch Phys Med Rehabil* 1985;66:592–597.

Jabre JF: Surface recording of the H reflex of the flexor carpi radialis. *Muscle & Nerve* 1981;4:435–438.

Jabre JF: Ulnar nerve lesions at the wrist: New techniques for recording from the sensory dorsal branch of the ulnar nerve. *Neurology* 1980;30:873–876.

Jebsen RH: Motor conduction velocity in proximal and distal segment of the radial nerve. *Arch Phys Med Rehabil* 1966;47:597–602.

Jimenez J, Easton JK, Redford JB: Conduction studies of the anterior and posterior tibial nerves. *Arch Phys Med Rehabil* 1970;51:164–169.

Johnson EW, Kukla RD, Wongsam PE: Sensory latencies to the ring finger: Normal values and relation to carpal tunnel syndrome. *Arch Phys Med Rehabil* 1981;62:206–208.

Johnson EW, Melvin JL: Sensory conduction studies of median and ulnar nerves. *Arch Phys Med Rehabil* 1967;48:25–30.

Johnson EW, Pease WS: *Practical electromyography*, 3rd ed. Baltimore: Williams & Wilkins, 1997:154–156.

Johnson EW, Sipski M, Lammertse T: median and radial sensory latencies to digit I: Normal values and usefulness in carpal tunnel syndrome. *Arch Phys Med Rehabil* 1987;68:140–141.

Kanakamedala RV, Hong CZ: Peripheral nerve entrapment at the knee localized by short segment stimulation. *Am J Phys Med Rehabil* 1989;68:116–122.

Kanakamedala RV, Simons DG, Porter RW, Zucker RS: Ulnar nerve entrapment at the elbow localized by short segment stimulation. *Arch Phys Med Rehabil* 1988;69:959–963.

Kaplan PE: Electrodiagnostic confirmation of long thoracic nerve palsy. *J Neurol Neurosurg Psychiatry* 1980;43:50–52.

Keesey JC: AAEM Minimonograph #33 Electrodiagnostic approach to defects of neuromuscular transmission. *Muscle & Nerve* 1989;12:613–626.

Kim DJ, Kalantri A, Guha S, Wainapel SF: Dorsal cutaneous nerve conduction: Diagnostic aid in ulnar neuropathy. *Arch Neurol* 1981;38:321–322.

Kimura J: *Electrodiagnosis in diseases of nerve and muscle: principles and practice*, 3rd ed. New York: Oxford University Press, 2001.

Kimura J: F-wave velocity in the central segment of the median and ulnar nerves. A study in normal subjects and in the patients with Charcot-Marie-Tooth disease. *Neurology (Minn)* 1974;24:539–546.

Kimura J, Bosch P, Linday GM: F-wave conduction velocity in the central segment of the peroneal and tibial nerves. *Arch Phys Med Rehab* 1975;56:492–497.

Kimura J: Principles and pitfalls of nerve conduction studies. *Ann Neurol* 1984;16:415–429.

Kimura J, Bodensteiner J, Yamada T: Electrically elicited blink reflex in normal neonates. *Arch Neurol* 1977;34:246–249.

Kimura J, Giron LT, Young SM: Electrophysiological study of Bell's palsy. Electrically elicited blink reflex in assessment of prognosis. *Arch Otolaryngol* 1976;102:140–143.

Kimura J, Powers JM, Van Allen MW: Reflex response of orbicularis oculi muscle to supraorbital nerve stimulation: Study in normal subjects and in peripheral facial paresis. *Arch Neurol* 1969;21:193–199.

Kimura I, Seiki H, Sasao SI, Ayyar DR: The greater auricular nerve conduction study: A technique, normative data and clinical usefulness. *Electromyogr Clin Neurophysiol* 1987;27:39–43.

Kincaid JC, Phillips ll LH, Daube JR: The evaluation of suspected ulnar neuropathy at the elbow. Normal conduction study values. *Arch Neurol* 1986;43:44–47.

Knezevic W, Bajada S: Peripheral autonomic surface potential: A quantitative technique for recording sympathetic conduction in man. *J Neurol Sci* 1985;67:239–251.

Kraft GH: Axillary, musculocuataneous and suprascapular nerve latency studies. *Arch Phys Med Rehabil* 1972;53:383–387.

Kraft GH, Johnson EW: *Proximal motor conduction and late response.* AAEM workshop, Boston, September 1986.

Lambert EH: Diagnostic value of electrical stimulation of motor nerves. *Electroencephalogr Clin Neurophysiol* 1962;14 (Suppl 22):9–16.

Lee HJ: Electrophysiologic evaluation of supraclavicular nerves. *Muscle & Nerve* 2004 (*in press*).

Lee HJ, Bach JR, DeLisa JA: Deep peroneal sensory nerve: Standardization in nerve conduction study. *Am J Phys Med Rehabil* 1990;69:126–127.

Lee HJ, Bach JR, DeLisa JA: Peroneal nerve motor conduction to the proximal muscles. an alternative approach to conventional methods. *Am J Phys Med Rehabil* 1997;76:197–199.

Lo Monaco M, Pasqua PG, Tonali P: Conduction studies along the accessory, long thoracic, dorsal scapular, and thoracodorsal nerves. *Acta Neurol Scand* 1983;68:171–176.

Lum PB, Kanakamedala R: Conduction of the palmar cutaneous branch of the median nerve. *Arch Phys Med Rehabil* 1986;67:805–806.

MacDonell RA, Cros D, Shahani BT: Lumbosacral nerve root stimulation comparing electrical with surface magnetic coil techniques. *Muscle & Nerve* 1992;15:885–890.

Mackenzie K, DeLisa JA: Determining the distal sensory latency of the superficial radial nerve in normal adult subjects. *Arch Phys Med Rehabil* 1981;62:31–34.

MacLean IC, Mattioni TA: Phrenic nerve conduction studies: A new technique and its application in quadriplegic patients. *Arch Phys Med Rehabil* 1991;62:70–72.

Ma DM, Liveson JA: *Laboratory reference for clinical neurophysiology.* Philadelphia: FA Davis, 1992:72–75.

Markand ON, Kincaid JC, Pourmand RA, et al. Electrophysiologic evaluation of diaphragm by transcutaneous phrenic nerve stimulation. *Neurology* 1984;34:604–614.

Maynard FM, Stolov WC: Experimental error in determination of nerve conduction velocity. *Arch Phys Med Rehabil* 1972;53:362–372.

McIntosh KA, Preston DC, Logigian EL: Short-segment incremental studies to localize ulnar nerve entrapment at the wrist. *Arch Neurol* 1998;50:303–305.

Melvin JL, Harris DH, Johnson EW: Sensory and motor conduction velocities in the ulnar and median nerves. *Arch Phys Med Rehabil* 1966;47:511–519.

Mysiew WJ, Colachis SClll: Electrophysiologic study of the anterior interosseous nerve. *Am J Phys Med Rehabil* 1988;67:50–54.

Nakano KK, Lundergan C, Okihiro MM: Anterior interosseous syndrome. *Arch Neurol* 1977;34:477–480.

Oh SJ: *Electromyography: neuromuscular transmission studies.* Baltimore: Williams & Wilkins, 1988.

Oh SJ, Sarala PK, Kuba T, Elmore RS: Tarsal tunnel syndrome: electrophysiological study. *Arch Neurol* 1979;5:327–330.

Palliyath SK: A technique for studying the greater auricular nerve conduction velocity. *Muscle & Nerve* 1984;7:232–234.

Pease WS, Lee HH, Johnson EW: Forearm median nerve conduction velocity in carpal tunnel syndrome. *Electromyogr Clin Neurophysiol* 1990;30:299–302.

Pribyle R, You SB, Jantra P: Sensory nerve conduction velocity of the medial antebrachial cutaneous nerve. *Electromyogr Clin Neurophysiol* 1979;19:41–46.

Raffaele R, Emery P, Palmeri A et al: Sensory nerve conduction velocity of the trigeminal nerve. *Electromyograph Clin Neurophysiol* 1987;27:115–117.

Roberts MM, Wertsch JJ, Park TA, Mazur A, Oswald TA: Selective activation of the flexor carpi ulnaris. *Muscle & Nerve* 1994; 17:1099.

Rodriquez AA, Simpson DM: AAEM Course E: Approach to the patient with bulbar symptoms—case illustrations, Minneapolis, 1996.

Rutkove SB: AAEM Minimonograph no. 14 The effects of temperature in neuromuscular electrophysiology. *Muscle & Nerve* 2001;24: 867–882.

Saadeh PB, Crisafulli CF, Bosner J, Wolf E: Needle electromyography of the diaphragm: a new technique. *Muscle & Nerve* 1993;16:15–20.

Saeed MA, Gatens PF: Compound nerve action potentials in the medial and lateral plantar nerves through tarsal tunnel. *Arch Phys Med Rehabil* 1982;63:304–307.

Schuchmann JA: Sural nerve conduction: A standardized technique. *Arch Phys Med Rehabil* 1977;58:166–168.

Schumm F, Stohr M: Accessary nerve stimulation in the assessment of myasthenia gravis. *Muscle & Nerve* 1984;7:147–151.

Shanker K, Means KM: Accessory nerve conduction in neck dissection subjects. *Arch Phys Med Rehabil* 1990;71:403–405.

Simpson JA: Fact and fallacy in measurement of conduction velocity in motor nerve. *J Neurol Neurosurg Psychiatry* 1964;27:381–385.

Siroky MB, Sax DS, Krane RJ: Sacral signal tracing: The electrophysiology of the bulbocavernosus reflex. *J Urol* 1979;122:661–664.

Spindler HA, Felsenthal G: Sensory conduction in the musculocutaneous nerve. *Arch Phys Med Rehabil* 1978;59:20–23.

Stevens JC: AAEM Course D: Practical suggestions for performing the needle electrode examination, Montreal, 1995.

Stevens JC: AAEM Minimonograph no. 26: the electrodiagnosis of carpal tunnel syndrome. *Muscle & Nerve* 1997;20:1477–1486.

Stomic A, Rosenfalck A, Buchthal F: Electrical and mechanical response of normal and myasthenic muscle with particular reference to the staircase phenomenon. *Brain Res* 1968;10:1–78.

Tonzola RF, Ackil AA, Shahani BT, Young RR: Usefulness of electrophysiological studies in the diagnosis of lumbosacral root disease. *Ann Neurol* 1981;9:305–308.

Trojaborg W, Sindrup EH: Motor and sensory conduction in different segments of the radial nerve in normal subjects. *J Neurol Neurosurg Psychiatry* 1969;32:354–359.

Waylonis GW, Johnson EW: Facial nerve conduction delay. *Arch Phys Med Rehabil* 1964;45:539–547.

Wertsch JJ: AAEM case report no. 25: anterior interosseous nerve syndrome. *Muscle & Nerve* 1992;15:977–983.

Yap CB, Hirota T: Sciatic nerve motor conduction velocity study. *J Neurol Neurosurg Psychiatry* 1967;30:233–239.

Index

Note: Page numbers in *italics* refer to illustrations.